# Arthritis and Rheumatism
## Your Questions Answered

By

**Dr Andrei Calin**
Consultant Rheumatologist,
Royal National Hospital for
Rheumatic Disease, Bath, UK

**Dr John Cormack**
General Practitioner, Greenwood
Surgery, Chelmsford, Essex, UK

CHURCHILL LIVINSTONE INTERNATIONAL
EDINBURGH LONDON MADRID MELBOURNE NEW YORK TOKYO 1996

CHURCHILL LIVINGSTONE INTERNATIONAL

Distributed in the United States of America by Churchill
Livingstone Inc., 650 Avenue of the Americas, New York, NY
10011, and by associated companies, branches and representatives
throughout the world.

First published 1996


ISBN 0443 049 882


**British Library Cataloguing in Publication Data**
A catalogue record for this book is available from the British Library

**Library of Congress Cataloging in Publication Data available**

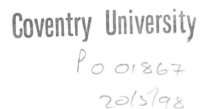

Printed and bound in Great Britain by
Biddles Ltd, Guildford and King's Lynn

# Contents

# Preface

The average general practitioner (GP) sees too many patients and has too little time and we know that some 20–30% of consultations relate to the locomotor system. Many GPs feel they have an inadequate exposure during their medical training focusing on rheumatological problems. Inevitably, if the practitioner had more information at his or her fingertips regarding everyday rheumatological conditions, life would be easier. The purpose of this book is to focus on common, everyday aches and pains of a rheumatological-medical orthopaedic nature. Common things commonly happen and that is why we are focusing on day-to-day occurrences in the hope that this text will help the practitioner listen to and manage the patient with rheumatic disorders. Above all, we hope that it will be read with enjoyment and that future patients who present with aches and pains will be anticipated with pleasure rather than the all too well recognized sinking feeling.

1996                                                                          A.C.

                                                                             J.C.

# 1. Introduction

Every general practitioner (GP) would expect to see at least a few patients each day with rheumatological problems. It is well recognized that around 20–30% of visits to the GP are in some way related to the locomotor system. One difficulty for many practitioners is that medical schools have failed to face up to reality, and it may well be that the average GP has received only a few hours of education in rheumatology and that often from an orthopaedic surgeon instead of a rheumatologist!

There are many reasons, apart from the mere prevalence of rheumatological disorders, that would make a practitioner want to know more about everyday rheumatology. For example, most rheumatological problems are easily dealt with in the GP's surgery and many patients can be treated satisfactorily by the practitioner with an interest in this speciality. Secondly, many patients with a rheumatological disorder, have a condition that lasts for decades rather than weeks and so the practitioner will have to have an understanding of the management of some of these often difficult to treat long-term problems. Thirdly, the linchpin in the GP–patient–specialist relationship must be the GP because it is the GP who will be managing day-to-day problems, some of which can be dramatic and potentially lethal. Inevitably, many anti-rheumatic drugs carry with them not only benefits but also side-effects, some of which may be life-threatening. The practitioner must be familiar with these potential hazards.

There are some 220 different rheumatological disorders recognized. Naturally, GPs will not need to be familiar with all, or even many, of these disorders. However, he or she must have a clear logical approach to the patient presenting with a rheumatological symptom. For example, should the patient simply be reassured that the problem is not serious? Should the patient be given a simple analgesic and told to return in a month? Should a non-steroidal anti-inflammatory drug (NSAID) be prescribed? Should the patient have some routine laboratory tests? Should a radiographic examination be performed? Should a physiotherapist be involved? Should the patient be referred to a rheumatologist or to an orthopaedic surgeon? How can the busy practitioner make a quick decision in each situation that arises? The purpose of this book is to direct the practitioner's train of thought in such a way that simple decisions can be made in many different situations.

Perhaps the greatest problems in rheumatological practice relate to over-investigation and over-treatment. It is very rare for a rheumatologist to see a patient who has been under-treated or under-investigated. One explanation for this is the relative lack of education as already mentioned. Another is that rheumatology is becoming ever more complicated, and is ever evolving, and it is sometimes difficult for the busy practitioner to keep abreast of the most recent developments.

In summary, an increase in knowledge about rheumatological problems will allow the GP to do much for many people, very quickly — usually at reasonable cost and quite simply. For example, reassurance may be enough to sort out the entire situation or a single, well-placed injection of corticosteroid may relieve months of suffering. Finally, it should be pointed out that few conditions are more confusing for the patient than rheumatological pain and stiffness. Many of the individuals arriving in the practice are fearful that they have a relentlessly progressive disorder that will end up with them in a wheelchair at best or bed-ridden at the worst. Education is clearly of paramount importance and here the GP is in the front line. Numerous publications from the Arthritis and Rheumatism Council, the National Osteoporosis Society, the National Ankylosing Spondylitis Society, the Lupus Society and other national institutions and patient-operated groups are helpful. The appendix includes the relevant telephone numbers and addresses that will help the practitioner in solving the many problems that arise in everyday practice.

# 2. General principles for diagnosing joint disease

In order to reach a diagnosis or at least a management plan it is necessary to take a history, examine the patient and, if necessary, carry out some simple laboratory and radiological studies. In general it is unnecessary to focus on many months or years of history and it is advantageous to have the patient report symptoms from the previous days rather than weeks or months. This allows the practitioner to focus on the major relevant problems. Following that, the examination may help and together with a history provide the diagnosis and treatment plan. It should always be appreciated that laboratory tests and radiological reports often confuse rather than clarify the picture and so reliance on these investigations may be inappropriate.

## 2.1 What is the current classification of joint disease?

Over 200 different types of arthritis are recognized. These range from degenerative to inflammatory, acute to chronic, monoarticular to polyarticular, and predominantly articular or extra-articular diseases. Inflammatory arthritis may be seropositive (i.e. rheumatoid arthritis, RA) or seronegative (i.e. viral, ankylosing spondylitis — AS, psoriatic arthropathy, etc.). The story is more complicated because although by definition, seropositive polyarthritis is RA, seronegative polyarthritis can occasionally evolve into seropositive disease or persist as a seronegative phenomenon. The latter, in turn, can be 'seronegative RA' or one of the other seronegative entities. Occasionally, polymyalgia rheumatica can have an inflammatory joint com-ponent and there are relative rarities such as polyarticular degenerative disease with a super-added inflammatory joint process.

3

**Table 2.1** Summary of the structures involved in common joint diseases

| Pathophysiological category | Prototypic disease | Number of sites | Typical sites | Systemic symptoms |
|---|---|---|---|---|
| Synovitis | Rheumatoid arthritis | Many | PIP, MCP, wrists | Yes |
| Enthesitis | Ankylosing spondylitis | One to many | Sacroiliac joints, spine | Rare |
| Microcrystalline arthritis | Gout | One | Great toe, knee | No |
| Cartilage degeneration | Osteoarthritis | One to many | DIP, hip, knee, spine | No |
| Infection | Staphylococcal arthritis | One | Knee | Yes |
| Focal injury | Low back pain | One | Variable | No |
| General conditions | Fibrositis | Many | Variable | No |
| Multisystem diseases | SLE | Many | Variable | Yes |

Inevitably, there is a variety of rare conditions ranging from haemochromatosis to viral hepatitis and other entities that can be associated with polysynovitis of varying degree.

## 2.2 What are the structures involved in joint disease?

Cartilage is primarily involved in the degenerative joint diseases (osteoarthritis — OA, or osteoarthrosis), whereas the synovium bears the brunt of the change in inflammatory arthritis (e.g. rheumatoid or infective arthritis).Within the synovial fluid, crystals are representative of gout (sodium urate crystals) or pseudogout (pyrophosphate crystal deposition). Pain at the insertion of the capsule into the joint (i.e. the site of the enthesis) is characteristic of the spondylarthropathies. To a varying degree, the 220 recognized rheumatological disorders all affect the joint or juxta-articular tissue either at single or multiple sites (Table 2.1).

## 2.3 What are the main extra-articular tissues involved in joint disease?

Any tissue anywhere can be involved as an extra-articular phenomenon in joint disorders. For example, although RA is a condition that focuses on the joints, there is also eye involvement (e.g. dry eyes, corneal ulcers), pulmonary disease (pulmonary

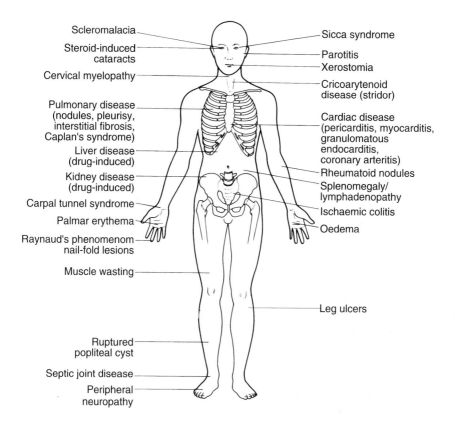

Sicca syndrome

Parotitis

Xerostomia

Cricoarytenoid disease (stridor)

Cardiac disease (pericarditis, myocarditis, granulomatous endocarditis, coronary arteritis)

Rheumatoid nodules

Splenomegaly/ lymphadenopathy

Ischaemic colitis

Oedema

Leg ulcers

Scleromalacia

Steroid-induced cataracts

Cervical myelopathy

Pulmonary disease (nodules, pleurisy, interstitial fibrosis, Caplan's syndrome)

Liver disease (drug-induced)

Kidney disease (drug-induced)

Carpal tunnel syndrome

Palmar erythema

Raynaud's phenomenom nail-fold lesions

Muscle wasting

Ruptured popliteal cyst

Septic joint disease

Peripheral neuropathy

**Fig. 2.1** The many extra-articular symptoms and signs in rheumatoid disease. Generalized symptoms include fatigue, fever, increased risk of infection, hyperviscosity syndrome, haematological abnormalities, Felty's syndrome, vasculitis, neuromuscular involvement, amyloidosis, osteoporosis, and drug toxicity.

fibrosis), vasculitis (affecting any tissue) and rheumatoid nodules (deposited anywhere), so that any specialist in medicine can be involved in the patient with rheumatoid disease. In fact all the connective tissue disorders are multisystem diseases in nature and both the GP and rheumatologist must be involved with every organ and every possible situation either as a primary event of the disease or as a side-effect of drug therapy (Fig. 2.1). Among the latter, for example, one may be dealing with gold nephropathy, methotrexate lung disease, non-steroidal induced gastric or duodenal ulceration and other phenomena.

## HISTORY, EXAMINATION AND SYMPTOMS

### 2.4  What is the importance of the patient's history?

A careful history is of paramount importance in helping the physician towards a diagnosis. The patient's personal and family history are of importance because, for example, an individual with relatives with psoriasis or AS may, in turn, have psoriatic arthropathy or one of the spondylarthropathies. RA also 'runs in families', though to a lesser extent. Contact with children with facial rash or viral-type illness may suggest a viral polysynovitis such as that seen associated with parvovirus.

However, if time is limited, as it usually is in general practice, then it is more beneficial to spend additional minutes examining the patient than to listen to a 20-year diary of events that will often be confusing. My approach is to focus on the symptoms over the last few days. However, it is worth stressing that we want to know whether the problem began suddenly over a few days (e.g. non-specific back pain) or slowly over weeks or months (e.g. AS).

### 2.5  What examination is appropriate when time is limited?

Time is always limited. I begin by examining the painful area, hoping that this will provide a quick answer. If there is no obvious local cause I then consider referred pain and perform a more detailed examination. Unfortunately, it is difficult to take a short cut and an examination of the whole body becomes necessary. For example, a patient with a swollen knee may have psoriatic arthritis and only by looking at the nails, umbilicus or gluteal cleft will the diagnosis be made. Alternatively, pain in the forearm may relate to the neck rather than local pathology at the elbow or wrist. Another point to remember is that the body has two sides and it is often helpful to compare the abnormal part with the contralateral normal side in order to discern whether there really is a difference. With the back examination, it is necessary to decide whether this alone will suffice or whether examination of the hip, trochanteric bursa, reflexes and power or other more peripheral phenomena is needed. If there is no leg pain and only back pain then usually examination can confined simply to the back. However, if there is leg pain, examination must include both the back and the leg.

## 2.6 What is synovitis?

Synovitis is inflammation of the synovium, which is normally two or three layers thick. The term is often used synonymously with arthritis. Following a variety of insults, the lining of the joint (the synovium) becomes thickened with many new layers of cells. New blood vessels develop within the tissue and the synovium proliferates until it can become a centimetre or more thick, as seen in some chronic cases of rheumatoid disease. The proliferating synovium produces more fluid than it absorbs and the joint becomes progressively thicker with both increasing synovium and synovial fluid.

## 2.7 In which diseases is synovitis a feature?

Synovitis is a feature of many primary inflammatory diseases such as RA itself, psoriatic arthritis, enteropathic arthropathy, bypass arthropathy and other entities. In addition, low-grade synovitis may be associated with degenerative joint disease, although the changes are often rather minimal. Infective synovitis may be caused by a range of infective agents from fungi to mycobacteria, Gram-positive and Gram-negative bacilli and cocci and viruses. Synovitis also occurs complicating leukaemic infiltrations, amyloid and crystal deposition diseases (e.g. urate/gout or pyrophosphate/pseudogout).

## 2.8 How do the synovitis-based illnesses present to the GP?

Synovitis may present acutely within a few hours or insidiously over months. For example, septic arthritis following staphylococcal or streptococcal infection, crystal synovitis (gout, pseudogout or other rarer crystal disorders) and reactive arthritis (from *Chlamydia*, or *Salmonella*, etc.) may present over hours. By contrast, the chronic arthritides such as RA, psoriatic arthropathy and other disorders tend to present more slowly over weeks or even months.

In general, monosynovitis tends to present acutely while polysynovitis is frequently more insidious in onset — but this is not always the case. For example, tubercular monoarthropathy can present slowly while rheumatoid polyarthritis can present overnight.

## 2.9  Is there a difference between synovitis in RA and in the other inflammatory diseases?

In RA the synovial biopsy reveals thickened fingers of tissue full of lymphocytes and even germinal centres, giving the classical pathology of rheumatoid disease. Interestingly, however, apart from these germinal centres, there are no definite qualitative differences between RA and the many other causes of an inflammatory synovitis. In fact, the differences are predominantly quantitative rather than qualitative.

## 2.10  If the patient presents with synovitis in a single joint, what does this suggest?

There are two major issues. First, one can see a patient who is followed long term with, for example, rheumatoid disease where he or she presents with a flare-up of symptoms in one joint. Such an individual should be considered to have a septic complication until proven otherwise. By contrast, the majority of individuals who attend the GP will have a local musculoskeletal problem, the most common sites being the shoulder, elbow or knee (see Chapters 5 and 6).

## 2.11  Which conditions present with polyarthralgia?

The two main entities are polymyalgia rheumatica and a variety of non-specific pain syndromes that include the so-called myofascial pain syndrome (i.e. fibromyalgia, and the old-fashioned label of 'fibrositis' — see Chapter 5). In fact, there is a third group that may present with a polyarthralgia picture or polyarthritis. Specifically, the viral disorders relating to parvovirus, influenza, rubella and other infections can give a mixture of arthralgia and arthritis.

## 2.12  If a patient presents with early morning stiffness but no other symptoms, what would this suggest?

Morning stiffness has always been a significant symptom in rheumatology. Indeed, it is an important criterion in the diagnosis of several inflammatory disorders.

In general, we understand little about morning stiffness although we recognize that patients with RA, psoriatic arthropathy, AS and other inflammatory arthropathies are likely to have stiffness, particularly in the morning and after rest. In addition, patients with degenerative arthropathy have stiffness but this is usually most prevalent after periods of exercise or sitting rather than specifically in the early morning. The duration of morning stiffness is also a useful variable to follow in managing the patient. It would be unusual to see a patient with active RA who has less than 30 or 60 minutes of morning stiffness, whereas it would be equally unusual to see a patient with degenerative arthropathy who has more than 10 minutes of morning stiffness. Furthermore, during treatment, as the disease becomes suppressed with an appropriate disease-modifying agent, the morning stiffness should improve, along with the improving laboratory variables.

### 2.13  How should a patient who presents with weakness and little or no pain be approached?

Weakness suggests a neurological or muscular problem rather than a primary rheumatological disorder. In general, a careful neurological evaluation will reveal the underlying cause of the problem and point the way to the appropriate management. Early referral to a neurologist may be needed.

## INVESTIGATIONS

### 2.14  Are laboratory investigations always required for diagnosis?

No! Many diagnoses are obvious from the history and examination. The main reasons for making a specific diagnosis in rheumatology include the need for specific therapy to be directed against a particular cause (e.g. sepsis or crystals) or to be able to educate the patient regarding the nature of the problem and the long-term outlook. Indeed, it is often comforting for the patient to have a specific label even if there is no specific therapy. However, therapy is often non-specific and much and energy should not be wasted defining a process, if treatment can settle the problem.

However, when assessing patients presenting with arthralgia, it is very helpful to know if you are dealing with a non-specific problem such as an unhappy individual who simply presents to the doctor with joint pains, headache or other non-specific entities, or whether there is an inflammatory disorder such as polymyalgia rheumatica. In such a patient, an erythrocyte sedimentation rate (ESR) or plasma viscosity will be elevated.

### 2.15  What is the role of synovial fluid examination?

If a patient presents with an acute monoarthritis then, ideally, synovial fluid should be removed in order to define the presence of crystals or infection. If a septic joint is suspected, referral to hospital is the norm where blood cultures should also be performed since it is often easier to culture the organism from blood than the joint. If the fluid appears sterile, careful examination of the genitourinary tract would be appropriate, looking for evidence of gonococcal disease in the urethra, vagina or cervix.

### 2.16  In general, what is the role of blood tests?

Blood tests are required either to help with a specific diagnosis or to test for safety in terms of potentially toxic drugs.

### 2.17  When should an erythrocyte sedimentation rate (ESR) or plasma viscosity test be performed?

In a patient presenting with general symptoms but no frank arthritis, a plasma viscosity or ESR is essential in indicating inflammatory activity. If these tests are abnormally elevated then there is a definite inflammatory disease such as RA or polymyalgia rheumatica, whereas if the results are negative, there is almost certainly a fibromyalgia or pain augmentation syndrome or other such entity. However, ESR and plasma viscosity are non-specific and may be raised in other conditions. Also, rarely, a patient with an inflammatory disorder may not have raised inflammatory indices.

### 2.18  How useful is the haemoglobin level when assessing a patient with a rheumatological complaint?

The haemoglobin level is often an indicator of disease activity and is a very useful monitor in chronic disease since active disease translates into a falling haemoglobin and vice versa. For example, a patient with RA and a history of joint disease for 5 years may well have the anaemia of chronic disease. If by contrast, the haemoglobin is normal, the disease can be assumed to be mild or in remission.

## 2.19  When should uric acid be measured?

If a patient presents with joint pains but no obvious acute, very painful, swollen joint it is entirely wrong to measure serum uric acid, because, regardless of what the urate reveals, the patient will not have gout. In fact, for every 50 individuals with hyperuricaemia, only one has gout! And remember, any patient on a diuretic is likely to have hyperuricaemia. In summary, hyperuricaemia alone is not a clear indication of a clinical gout.

In a patient with proven gout, the serum urate measurement is helpful where allopurinol is used and may be repeated on one or two occasions to see whether the uric acid production is being suppressed by the therapy. If the uric acid remains stubbornly high, it should be assumed that there has been poor compliance before automatically increasing the dosage.

## 2.20  What is the role of rheumatoid factor?

Rheumatoid factor is always helpful in differentiating whether a patient has synovitis of the seropositive RA type or one of the other inflammatory arthritides, e.g. AS or psoriatic arthropathy. However, if a patient presents with odd joint aches but no frank arthritis it is usually unhelpful to measure rheumatoid factor. Thus, a patient with arthralgias and seropositivity for rheumatoid factor almost certainly does not have RA whereas a patient with polysynovitis that looks like 'RA' but is seronegative for rheumatoid factor probably does not have RA. A search for psoriasis and other entities should be made.

In general, it should be remembered that some 5–10% of the normal population are seropositive for rheumatoid factor whereas RA itself occurs in well under 1% of the population. Put another way, no more than 10% of individuals who are seropositive for rheumatoid factor actually have RA. Thus, it is of paramount importance to dovetail the laboratory results with the history and clinical findings.

## 2.21 How useful is assessment of the anti-nuclear factor (ANF) status?

In a patient with multisystem disease, a positive ANF is very help-ful in directing attention towards systemic lupus erythematosus (SLE). However, ANF positivity may be present in some 3–4% of the population while SLE occurs only in 1 in 1000 individuals. Thus, the majority of ANF-positive individuals do not have SLE.

## 2.22 Is the HLA B27 test useful?

HLA B27 testing has virtually no role in general practice. Although over 95% of patients with AS are HLA B27 positive, it must be remembered that some 8% of the normal population also carry this antigen. It is therefore wrong to request HLA B27 in the assessment of a patient with back pain. If the story is sugges-tive of AS (i.e. (1) insidious onset of back pain; (2) coming on in an individual around the age of 20 or 30 years; (3) with an associ-ation with morning stiffness; (4) showing improvement with exer-cise; (5) persistence of symptoms for over 3 months) there are good grounds to request a pelvic radiograph. If sacroiliitis is pre-sent the patient has AS. If, by contrast, the sacroiliac joints are normal then the patient does not have AS, regardless of the HLA B27 status.

## 2.23 What is the role of radiology in diagnosis?

Many forms of arthropathy are associated with normal radio-graphs in terms of bone and cartilage structure. However, there may be evidence of soft-tissue swelling or synovial fluid but this is more readily recognized clinically rather than by radiography. There are a few characteristic radiological changes. However, radiographic examinations should be performed sparingly (in order to save the patient unnecessary time, trouble, expenses and irradiation) and it should be borne in mind that radiographic findings do not always correlate well with symptoms. For exam-ple, a radiograph of a knee showing OA might lead one to expect that nothing can be done — whereas the reverse is often the case (e.g. the symptoms are caused by weak muscles, ligamentous damage, etc., and can be readily treated, whereas the 'OA' is irrelevant and does not require treatment).

## 2.24  What are the characteristic radiological changes in joint disease?

- *RA* may reveal the classical erosions associated with juxta-articular osteoporosis, cartilage loss (i.e. joint-space narrowing) and joint deformity. In particular, rheumatoid disease typically affects small and large joints alike in a symmetrical distribution.
- *Degenerative arthropathy* may show osteophytosis, juxta-articular sclerosis, cartilage loss, occasional bone cysts and joint deformity. Degenerative joint disease typically affects the distal interphalangeal joints of the hands, the first carpometacarpal joint, the hips and the knees. Strikingly, the ankles are spared.
- *Chronic gout* may reveal large rat-bite like erosions particularly around the first MTP joint. However, most patients with gout have normal radiography.
- *Chondrocalcinosis* defines the situation where crystals of calcium pyrophosphate deposit in hyaline and fibrocartilage. This is usually a chance radiological finding but may be associated with acute pseudogout because the pyrophosphate crystals cause inflammation.
- *Psoriatic arthropathy* destroys bone more than cartilage and there may be what is known as acro-osteolysis whereby the distal ends of the small long bones in the hands become eroded giving a pencil-in-cup appearance. It is a relatively localized oligoarticular condition that is patchy in nature and often asymmetrical.
- *AS and the other spondylarthritides* result in sacroiliitis — by definition in 100% of patients with AS and perhaps in 20% of those with secondary forms of spondylarthropathy (i.e. related to psoriasis, inflammatory bowel disease or Reiter's disease).
- *Acute infective arthritis* typically reveals no change apart from some osteoporosis but, as the untreated arthropathy progresses, there may be marked destruction.
- *Fungal or tubercular arthropathy*, being insidious in nature, will show more obvious long-term damage with bone collapse, osteonecrosis and other changes.
- *Diffuse idiopathic skeletal hyperostosis* is typically a chance radiological finding. The proliferative bone formation is wax-like in appearance and is typically symptom-free. It is rarely of clinical significance.

- *Spondylolisthesis,* a forward slippage of one vertebra on the next, seen on the radiograph to a minor extent, is usually of no importance. Spinal instability *per se* is very unusual. Of course there are the rare exceptions with gross degrees of instability but this usually relates to major trauma or major developmental anomalies and would be treated surgically.

For patients with multisystem rheumatological disorders, a chest radiograph and other investigations may be required.

## PRACTICAL PROBLEMS IN DIAGNOSIS

### 2.25 How should I approach the problem of the patient who hurts all over?

Unfortunately, this situation is all too common. The question can only be answered if you know the background of the clinical situation. At one end of the spectrum is the patient who presents to the GP having seen no doctor before. The complaint is that he or she hurts all over. At the other end of the spectrum is the patient who has already seen other specialists, and almost certainly has a variety of diagnostic labels ranging from 'there is nothing wrong' to 'ME' (myalgic encephalomyelitis), to myofascial pain syndrome (i.e. fibromyalgia), a psychological functional disorder, etc. The options for the first patient would be different from those for the second!

The approach must be to take the history and to examine the patient. A new patient will require some very simple investigations, such as a full blood picture and plasma viscosity or ESR, to be performed. The patient already investigated almost certainly requires no more tests, having probably received numerous radiographs, invasive tests, blood tests, etc. already.

If the initial ESR or plasma viscosity is elevated then polymyalgia rheumatica (Chapter 5) may be present. The latter typically causes proximal upper limb and lower limb discomfort rather than 'pain all over'. The most important point of all, therefore, is to ascertain from the patient whether the pain is really 'all over' or whether there is one major and worse area, since if this can be treated (e.g. an injection into the shoulder) then the confidence of the patient will rise and with that the entire problem will more readily be defused.

Patients at both ends of the spectrum require understanding and a sympathetic approach but the sympathy must be married to an aggressive, optimistic and determined treatment programme, most probably through referral to a rheumatologist with the necessary interest, skills and sensitivity to deal with such a patient.

In summary, if the patient has a specific clearly defined disease such as polymyalgia rheumatica the issue is quite straightforward (Chapter 5). By contrast, for the patient with a non-specific problem such as those with the various labels introduced above, much more time and energy is required. However, it is quite clear that an investment in time and energy early on will solve a lot of trouble in the long term. Certainly, the patient with generalized pains is an appropriate referral and no GP should feel that the rheumatologist's time is being 'wasted' simply because there is nothing to find on examination or with the laboratory tests.

## 2.26 How should I deal with the patient who presents with a rheumatological condition superimposed on other pathologies?

It is always important to avoid preconceived ideas. The patient may be certain that they have disease 'A' and it is important not to be steamrollered into the wrong direction, since 'A' may be part of the problem but with a superimposed second disorder, the relative contribution of the two can sometimes only be disentangled with difficulty.

You should therefore spend less time listening to the patient and more time performing an examination. In general, it takes much longer to listen to a poor historian recount many different and often inappropriate slants of the story while, by contrast, a quick but careful examination may rapidly reveal the nature of the aetiology and pathology.

## 2.27 What should I do if a patient presents with a history of trauma but in whom I suspect a systemic problem?

This can be a very difficult situation. For example, a patient may arrive with a very clear story of a traumatic insult to, for example, the knee. This settles only very little over the ensuing weeks and you are then presented with what could be a post-traumatic effusion or a coincidental episode of trauma with a self-limiting problem but now with a superimposed reactive or other form of arthropathy. Clearly, a detailed history searching for other symptoms (e.g. diarrhoea, skin lesions, urethritis, photophobia, etc.) and a careful examination in search of other signs (e.g. silent mouth ulcers, clinically silent balanitis, keratoderma blenorrhagia, etc.) will be required to establish the possibility of a secondary disorder. Laboratory tests may help in addition. Certainly an ESR or plasma viscosity would be appropriate.

## 2.28  What if I have difficulty in reaching a diagnosis?

In general, the disease will evolve into a more clearly defined entity and it matters little if a few weeks have been lost before attaching the appropriate label. For example, a patch of psoriasis may appear, or the patient may begin to develop diarrhoea, revealing the underlying diagnosis of psoriatic arthropathy on the one hand or enteropathic disease on the other.

In the rare example of individuals with leukaemic infiltration, there is also widespread metastatic disease elsewhere and missing the diagnosis by a few weeks will not have any major impact on outcome. Of course, the opposite is the case with infective arthritis but it would be entirely unreasonable to carry out a synovial biopsy and culture in every patient presenting with a monoarthritis. The odd case of tuberculosis may always be missed for at least a few weeks until radiological change occurs or other factors emerge. Clearly in a case that does not resolve it may be worthwhile getting help from a rheumatologist.

## 2.29  What are the common misdiagnoses?

A major pitfall would be the introduction of corticosteroid therapy by mouth unless it is certain that you are dealing with a self-limiting post-viral phenomenon since corticosteroids are effectively contraindicated in RA unless all else has failed.

Another diagnostic pitfall is that of mislabelling an erosive inflammatory degenerative arthropathy (nodal generalized osteoarthritis) as RA. The former occurs in the older population in whom seropositivity for rheumatoid factor is more prevalent than in younger individuals. This is a chance laboratory finding since rheumatoid factor is present in some 5% of normal individuals. Again, relying too strongly on laboratory findings can be misleading.

A common mistake is for a patient with reactive arthritis or Reiter's disease to be wrongly diagnosed as having gonococcal arthropathy and given intravenous penicillin. Not surprisingly, the arthropathy does not improve!

Hyperuricaemia does not mean gout! A patient with a painful joint and hyperuricaemia may have an infection and diet- or diuretic-related hyperuricaemia.

### 2.30  How can I tell if chest wall pain is caused by costochondritis?

Firstly there should be a high index of suspicion that this could be the cause. Too often patients have been referred to the cardiologist, chest physician or even psychologist rather than to a rheumatologist. The important point is that the pain is often diffuse and poorly localized by the patient but close inspection will reveal the classical trigger sites at the anterior chest wall joints (costochondral) or posterior chest wall (costovertebral). Usually only two or three joints are affected and local steroid injections can solve the problem. Equally important, strong reassurance that there is no underlying cardiac or pulmonary disease will benefit the patient. Also, remember that posterior chest wall disease may be associated with pain that radiates anteriorly or vice versa.

### 2.31  Does menopausal arthritis exist?

There is no evidence that a clearly defined separate entity labelled as 'menopausal arthritis' exists, although clearly there are problems seen predominantly in women after the menopause, such as an increasing risk of osteoporosis and fracture and worsening degenerative joint disease. However, the change from normal hormonal status to menopausal levels does not appear to be associated with any exacerbation or amelioration of existing rheumatological disorders. Some diseases, such as polymyalgia rheumatica and giant cell arteritis, occur more commonly after the menopause but this would appear to be an age-related phenomenon since there is no difference in age of onset between men and women for these disorders. Gout can occur in women below the menopause but is certainly much more likely in the older female but again this does not appear to have an important hormonal influence.

### 2.32 What impact does a multiracial society have on the diagnosis?

No longer can the GP or rheumatologist simply assume that common things commonly happen! The physician must now accept that what would otherwise be an extraordinarily rare condition in a UK population of 'Anglo-Saxon' background, may now turn up with alarming frequency.

For example, a patient presenting with a swollen knee has a variety of possible aetiologies. However, a traveller or recent arrival from the Indian subcontinent may have tubercular joint disease! Similar comments can be made regarding rickets and osteomalacia — conditions that are rare in the indigenous population but more frequently seen in those with pigmented skin, much clothing and 'poor' diet, particularly in the north of the country where the short winter days may contribute further to the problem.

## EMERGENCIES REQUIRING IMMEDIATE REFERRAL

### 2.33 What emergency problems will I face for which immediate referral is mandatory?

There is a variety of acute medical emergencies in rheumatology. These situations require immediate referral to a rheumatologist or immediate initiation of therapy:

1. The acute monoarthropathy presenting over hours is either due to sepsis or to crystal synovitis until proven otherwise. The immediate steps must include joint aspiration and if necessary blood cultures followed by appropriate treatment. As the question implies, these cases are normally best dealt with in hospital.
2. The patient with chronic disease such as RA who suddenly develops a wrist drop, for example, may have an acute vasculitis and emergency referral is required for the initiation of high-dose corticosteroid and other suppressive therapy within hours rather than days.
3. A patient with chronic rheumatoid disease and scleromalacia may suddenly develop perforation of the lens with catastrophic

consequences. Such a problem should be assessed urgently by an ophthalmologist and rheumatologist.

4. Patients with giant cell arteritis/polymyalgia rheumatica may present with sudden loss of vision or rapid onset of general features of malaise, arthralgias and myalgias. Regardless of where the patient fits on the spectrum, an urgent ESR must be performed. Before the results return, high-dose corticosteroid must be initiation with at least 1 mg per kg of body weight, particularly if there is anything to suggest pain in and around the eye, blood vessel tenderness over the temporal arteries, deteriorating vision or other manifestations of giant cell arteritis. Clearly, early discussion with the rheumatologist will be necessary to confirm the diagnosis and determine the long-term management programme.

5. A patient presenting with acute onset calf swelling is often wrongly diagnosed as having a deep vein thrombosis. It is always important to establish whether there has been any knee synovitis and pain preceding the onset of calf pain and discomfort. At least in rheumatological practice, the commonest cause of calf pain is a ruptured popliteal cyst associated with the arthropathy. This can happen at any time. Unfortunately, casualty officers at hospital are often unaware of this common phenomenon and will instigate anticoagulant therapy, possibly with catastrophic results. If the diagnosis is wrong, bleeding can occur into the already inflamed calf. A high index of suspicion is needed to recognize a ruptured popliteal cyst. The patient may mention that the somewhat tender knee is now less swollen as the calf has become acutely more so. Intra-articular corticosteroid treatment into the knee is an excellent way of managing the symptoms quickly.

6. There is a group of miscellaneous and somewhat rare indications for acute management and these would include deteriorating renal failure in a patient with SLE and a variety of other complications of the less frequently occurring connective tissue disorders.

7. In a patient with long-standing rheumatoid disease, the spinal cord is always at risk from compression in the cervical spine. Thus, any patient with rheumatoid disease who suddenly develops long track signs with weakness in the lower limbs, bladder dysfunction, increasing neck pain and perhaps pain radiating down the arms, must have an urgent assessment by neurologist or rheumatologist. In such an individual, urgent

neurosurgical decompression may be indicated.

8. A patient with ankylosing spondilitis may present with photophobia and decoriating vision associated with a red eye. Such an individual needs urgent care from an ophthalmologist.

9. Regrettably, one of the commonest emergencies in rheumatological practice relates not to the underlying disease itself but rather to the toxicity of anti-rheumatic drugs. The story regarding NSAID-induced massive gastrointestinal bleeds is well known and particular attention should be paid to those individuals who are most at risk: older women with a past history of gastrointestinal discomfort or bleed as discussed in Chapter 11. In addition, the disease-suppressive agents such as gold, penicillamine, azathioprine and cyclophosphamide can cause sudden bone marrow toxicity while methotrexate may be associated with rapid-onset pulmonary failure. There must always be a high index of suspicion that any new symptom occurring in a patient with rheumatic disease has a drug-induced aetiology rather than being an exacerbation of the underlying disorder.

In summary, the practical advice is to retain a high index of suspicion and, if in doubt, refer to hospital immediately.

# 3. Neck pain

Patients frequently present with neck pain. It is helpful for the physician to think of neck pain in the same way that he would think of 'headache' — in most individuals pain relates to poor posture and muscle tension rather than sinister underlying pathology. It should be remembered that radiological change in the neck is common after the age of 20 years and undue reliance on the radiograph or radiology report should be avoided lest the architecture be blamed for what in fact is a muscle or ligament problem. Careful examination is usually more helpful than radiographic evaluation and laboratory tests have little or no role in the assessment of most patients with neck pain.

Perhaps the most important aspect of treatment is for the patient to realize that movement is almost always preferable to rest. Collars should almost always be avoided. Unless a patient has a dramatic degree of bone and joint destruction as seen in the occasional patient with rheumatoid arthritis (RA), little damage can occur from normal movement.

## 3.1 What are the common causes of neck pain?

Neck pain is extraordinarily common. In most people with neck pain there is no radiological evidence of any sinister underlying architectural/bone disease. In fact, as with most headaches, the usual cause of neck pain is muscle tension and tightness, and this may relate to the muscles or ligaments in the mid zones of the neck or to pain radiating down into the neck from the occiput or up into the neck from the periscapular musculature — particularly the rhomboids, trapezius muscle and the sternocleidomastoid muscle.

The patient may rapidly enter a vicious cycle: movement causes pain and therefore the head and neck stop moving. Often a bad posture is adopted and this increases the tension in the muscles and therefore increases the pain. For example, neck pain is commonly seen in musicians who concentrate for hours on music practice, and in office workers who do not sit correctly when typing.

A more uncommon cause of neck pain is an acute torticollis, whereby after sleeping in an uncomfortable position the patient wakes with sudden onset of pain in the neck, usually associated with a tilt to one or other side and difficulty in moving the neck because of the pain. Poor posture then tends to cause increasing pain and, unless the cycle can be interrupted quickly, the acute problem may become chronic. Also at night, the use of more than one pillow may result in neck pain if the head is kept in an very tilted position.

Pain can also relate to nerve root entrapment; for example, the C5/6 nerve root may be irritated by discogenic or osteophytic material in the lower neck. In such cases, the pain radiates down either shoulder into the upper and sometimes lower arm.

### 3.2  How does neck pain present?

In acute torticollis the patient will develop sudden pain; however, the most common situation is for a patient to present with insidious onset of pain over weeks rather than minutes or hours. This sort of pain is analogous to a headache in terms of an absence of obvious precipitating events. The patient may complain of pain on extremes of movement or, more typically, pain at the cervicothoracic junction.

One complicating feature is that once pain has become chronic over a few weeks, there is often spread of the symptoms (and signs) to other trigger sites and the patient may well develop a more generalized pain augmentation/fibromyalgic syndrome (see Chapter 5).

If the C5/6 nerve roots are involved (a rare event) the patient may present with nerve root irritation and dysaesthesiae (numbness and tingling) in the distribution of the nerve. For example, if C5/6 is the root involved then the thumb and index finger may develop some numbness and tingling while if C6/7 or C7/T1 are involved then the little finger and forearm will develop pain over the ulnar distribution. If the symptoms persist, there may be impulse pain with increased discomfort going down the upper limb on coughing or sneezing and this may be followed by weakness and increasing numbness. Reflex changes may follow (i.e. loss of triceps jerk, for example, in cases of C7 nerve root entrapment).

## 3.3 How should the patient with neck pain be examined?

As intimated above, most patients with neck pain have 'mechanical' rather than inflammatory, traumatic or other destructive aetiologies.

On examination there may well be decreased mobility, specifically, with pain arising from forward flexion, lateral flexion or rotation in either direction. This will establish to some degree where the trigger for the pain may be. Secondly, direct palpation for tenderness over the occipital crest, over the mastoid processes at the site of insertion of the sternocleidomastoid muscles, the interspinous ligament sites, usually between C5 and 6 and C6 and 7, and painful triggers at the proximal end of the musculature over the dorsal spines or medial border of the scapula are searched for. Also, the physician should note whether the posture is good or bad.

In individuals with nerve root involvement, cervical spine films would be required, perhaps with oblique views to get a closer look at the nerve foramina. Osteophytes may be seen causing a decreased area within which the nerve can freely move. Such an individual may respond to analgesics and a few days in a collar followed by gentle remedial exercises. However, if symptoms persist for 6 weeks or progress rapidly or are severe with a progressive neurodeficit, then an MRI scan would be appropriate with a view to neurosurgical referral and intervention.

## 3.4 What is the role of radiography?

The danger with taking a radiograph of the neck is that it will often show some form of 'arthritis' in the spine; indeed virtually everybody over the age of 25 years has some degenerative change. When patients learn that there is 'arthritis of the neck' (which they know is 'incurable') they may assume they will have neck pain for ever.

The reality is that most neck pain is soft tissue in origin, secondary to muscle and ligamentous problems and needs to be treated with the right exercises, with advice about a pillow, perhaps local injection and perhaps an NSAID.

The underlying architecture of the bone is probably irrelevant. Therefore, it may be best to avoid requesting the radiographic examination in the first place.

### 3.5  What are the main factors in the management of neck pain?

Treatment should be directed towards education and postural exercises, and if necessary anti-inflammatory treatment of the trigger site.

Education, as well as explanation and reassurance, is the most important aspect of management. Using the analogy of the common headache the patient should understand that the trouble emanates from the tense musculature rather than any sinister intrinsic pathology. In general, the physician should try to reassure patients that they do not need a radiograph unless there is evidence of possibility of fracture or obvious nerve root entrapment, perhaps by osteophytes.

The patient should be advised that, in general, movement is better than rest. If the neck 'rests' for more than 48 hours in a collar a vicious cycle may develop. Muscles that do not move become stiff and therefore hurt more and, in turn, posture deteriorates and thereafter any movement causes more pain, etc.

The patient should return to normal spinal mobility and, with this in mind, should be advised to decrease the pain in the short term with ice-packs or heat and thereafter to carry out an exercise programme. Perhaps, some 80% of patients find an ice-pack preferable, while 20% prefer a hot-water bottle. Alternatively, a hot shower may help decrease the pain sufficiently to allow the stretching and strengthening exercise programme to begin.

Attention to posture is of paramount importance. Patients should be encouraged to pay attention to posture at all times, for example, by leaving memos around the home and at work to remind themselves of the need for good posture and mobility.

At night, large pillows should be avoided as they push the head into lateral flexion and this abnormal posture during the night will create pain during the day. Only one small pillow is needed. In fact, any small support should be just tucked under the neck to maintain a relatively flat posture during the night.

Finally, my approach as a rheumatologist is to inject the painful trigger sites either at the interspinous space between C5 and 6 or C6 and 7 or at the scapula or occipital margins including the mastoid processes. Many GPs would prefer perhaps to manage with analgesics or NSAIDs, in addition to the exercises mentioned.

In general it is preferable to try to make patients' lives less complicated and to avoid unnecessary cost where possible. For example, for those with severe intractable head, neck and shoulder pain an inflatable halo cushion support may be appropriate. For most individuals, a very small pillow or even a rolled up towel can just fill the angle between the head, neck and shoulder, giving sufficient support at night.

## 3.6  What are the main exercises for neck pain?

For neck pain arising from the periscapular musculature, the patient should first be asked to shrug their shoulders right back whereby the scapulae are drawn towards each other. At the same time the chin should be slightly lowered to maintain a neutral or minimally flexed position and then the chin tucked in while the head is pushed back. This results in a more or less vertical position with the weight of the head supported by the shoulders; in this position the patient should be asked to count to five slowly and then relax completely back into their normal position. The procedure should then be repeated ten times, each for five seconds (i.e. one minute in total). This is repeated three or four times per day. Patients may find it helpful to stand directly against the wall, bringing their shoulder blades back towards the wall and also touching the wall with the occiput still keeping the chin tucked in.

For individuals with pain on moving or limitation of neck movement — for instance when trying to reverse their car — rotational and flexion exercises are appropriate. First, the neck should be flexed slightly — again tucking in the chin and rotating slowly to look over their right shoulder. When they can no longer move they should try and rotate an extra 0.5 cm and count to five slowly returning to the midline, and then to look over the contralateral shoulder. Again, when they reach the extreme of movement they should try and go just that extra few millimetres, hold it for 3 s and return to the neutral position repeating this procedure in each direction 10 times. Then, again with slight flexion, they should flex laterally the ear towards the shoulder ensuring that they do not cheat by lifting the shoulder to the ear. Once more, when the extreme is reached, they should try to go through the barrier, hold it for 3 s, slowly return to the neutral position and repeat the procedure to the contralateral side. The routine again is repeated on 10 occasions three times during the day.

It is worth telling the patient that, however tiresome these exercises sound, they will almost certainly be gratified by the rapid improvement. As so often happens, activities that the patients can do for themselves to improve their condition are the most satisfying for all concerned.

### 3.7  How should patients be managed if pain persists despite conservative management?

If neurosurgery is inappropriate, it may be necessary to give a cervical spine epidural injection in the same way that an epidural injection is given in the lumbar spine. This is frequently carried out by an anaesthetist, or other specialist running a pain clinic.

## TRAUMA

### 3.8  What are the common traumatic causes of neck pain?

Trauma is very rarely a cause for neck pain. However, much is spoken and written about 'whiplash' injuries. Individuals who are struck from behind in a road traffic accident are sprung forward, the neck being hyperextended on returning via the neutral position to the position of extension. Inevitably, this injury can result in neck pain. However, insurance, medicolegal and other complicating factors may come into play, and it is often difficult or impossible to dissect out what is residual neck pain relating to ongoing effects of the trauma and to what degree the persistent symptoms relate to stress, anxiety, compensation concerns, legal encouragement/interference and other factors.

Otherwise, the neck is relatively well protected and there are few 'common' traumatic causes apart from the occasional rugby or other contact-sport injury.

### 3.9  What particular features should be sought in traumatic neck pain?

There will be a clear history of trauma and the important first step is to define whether there is any neurological deficit. Specifically, the patient must be assessed for long track signs in the history (i.e. lower limb weakness, bowel or bladder dysfunction and other comparable major events) and, more locally, evidence of nerve root damage in the upper limb with pain radiating down to the hands, weakness and dysaesthesiae. Alteration in reflexes may also be found.

### 3.10 How should traumatic neck pain be managed in patients with ankylosing spondylitis ?

Normally, management will depend on the severity but, if there is any doubt, appropriate radiological assessment must be made. There is one important caveat. Patients with AS in whom fusion of the cervical spine has occurred, may sustain a cervical spine fracture after only minimal injury and in such individuals it is important to have a low threshold of suspicion for the consideration of nerve root or cord damage; in addition, particular attention should be paid to the radiological evaluation in order to define the presence or otherwise of bony injury. In such individuals, the injury may occur through the body of C6 or C7 and be missed on conventional views. If there is any possibility of such an injury, additional views should be taken through the axillary (or swimmer's) view and fracture of the lower cervical spine will then be seen. Naturally, transportation of any patient from the site of injury to the emergency room must be managed carefully, ensuring no movement of the head and neck.

### 3.11 When should a patient be referred?

If in doubt, refer. Clearly any chance of nerve or cord damage must be treated as an emergency. Long tract signs are of major significance. Pain alone is unlikely to be caused by a serious problem.

# 4. Back pain

In patients presenting with back pain, the first step is to distinguish between mechanical and inflammatory aetiologies. The main distinguishing features of history and examination are listed here. The inflammatory diseases are described in Chapters 7 and 9.

## 4.1 What are the features that distinguish between the mechanical and inflammatory aetiologies of back pain?

The patient may well have been to a variety of different individuals ranging from chiropractitioners to osteopaths and perhaps to other GPs, who may have given a diagnosis. However, it is important to begin with a clinical history followed by an examination.

A summary of the main features of history and examination that differentiate between mechanical and inflammatory causes of back pain are shown in Tables 4.1 and 4.2. Inflammatory back pain is discussed in Chapter 7, which includes the common non-infective inflammatory sacroiliitis associated with AS, and the more unusual presentation of septic sacroiliitis, which is seen typically in children under 10 years of age.

## 4.2 What is the place of radiography in the diagnosis of back pain?

In general, for every 100 radiographs of the spine that are requested, only one is relevant. As stressed elsewhere, the great problem with radiological evaluation is the lack of correlation between what the radiologist sees and reports and the pathology

**Table 4.1** Differential history in back symptoms of the mechanical and inflammatory type

|                              | Mechanical         | Inflammatory                |
|------------------------------|--------------------|-----------------------------|
| Past history                 | ±                  |                             |
| Family history               | –                  | +                           |
| Onset                        | Acute              | Insidious                   |
| Age (years)                  | 15–90              | < 40                        |
| Sleep disturbance            | ±                  | ++                          |
| Morning stiffness            | +                  | +++                         |
| Involvement of other systems | –                  | +                           |
| Effect of exercise           | Worse              | Better                      |
| Effect of rest               | Better             | Worse                       |
| Radiation of pain            | Anatomical (Sl, L5)| Diffuse (thoracic) buttock) |
| Sensory symptoms             | +                  | –                           |
| Motor symptoms               | +                  | –                           |

**Table 4.2** Differential findings on examination between back pain of mechanical and inflammatory type

|                      | Mechanical      | Inflammatory  |
|----------------------|-----------------|---------------|
| Scoliosis            | +               | –             |
| Range of movement decreased | Asymmetrically | Symmetrically |
| Local tenderness     | Local           | Diffuse       |
| Muscle spasm         | Local           | Diffuse       |
| Straight leg raising | Decreased       | Normal        |
| Sciatic nerve stretch| Positive        | Absent        |
| Hip involvement      | –               | +             |
| Neurodeficit         | +               | –             |
| Others systems       | –               | +             |

causing the symptoms. The physician must know that virtually everyone over the age of 20 or 25 years has some degenerative change in the spine. However, most people with evidence of osteophytosis, spondylosis, disc-space narrowing and other changes, are symptom-free. Apart from clear evidence of sacroiliitis or infection, a spinal vertebral collapse, fractures or local malignancy, there are few radiological changes that are relevant. A summary of the characteristic radiological changes in joint disease are listed in Q2.24.

Frequently, the GP states that it is patient-led pressure that persuaded him or her to request a radiograph. This is understandable but better education should in turn persuade the patient that radiographs are rarely indicated. My approach is merely to obtain a radiographic examination to confirm sacroiliitis or to help when conservative treatment modalities have failed. Another issue frequently raised is that of the medicolegal situation. Again, it can readily be argued that a radiograph should only be performed in fairly clearly defined situations. For example, if there is evidence of nerve root irritation and neurosurgical intervention is considered, a CT scan or MRI will be required in addition to the plain film.

Interestingly, in the USA, a patient will often quiz the GP on why the radiograph is needed. They will be concerned about the extra time needed to get a radiograph, they will be unhappy about the inevitable cost either in personal or societal terms and they are worried about the potential risk of unnecessary radiation. This rather healthy state of affairs translates into both patient and physician being more thoughtful before ordering any test.

## 4.3 What other investigations should be sought?

In general, blood tests should not be used as a screening investigation for back pain. For example, even with inflammatory spinal disease such as AS, the erythrocyte sedimentation rate (ESR) is frequently normal. In those patients presenting with widespread spinal pain and in whom GPs are concerned that multiple myeloma may be the cause (an exceptionally rare situation), a plasma viscosity or ESR would clearly be of great benefit.

However, in general, attention to the recent history and physical examination is more helpful than radiographs and blood tests. Further investigations should be considered as a last resort, and then usually in conjunction with the specialist (rheumatological or neurosurgical).

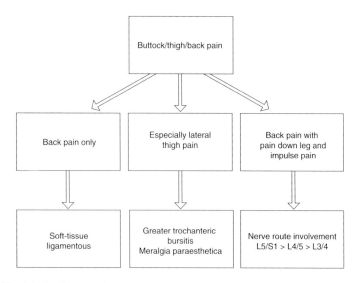

**Fig. 4.1** Algorithm showing the main categories of mechanical/ligamentous back pain.

## MECHANICAL/LIGAMENTOUS BACK PAIN

### 4.4 How is mechanical/ligamentous back pain categorized?

The first division is duration of pain, whether it has persisted for more or less than 6 weeks. Pain that has been present for under 6 weeks may well be self-limiting and can often be ignored. Once this cut-off point is passed, it makes little difference whether symptoms have been present for 2 months or 20 years. The search for the right diagnosis will be the same.

Secondly, it is necessary to establish whether there is nerve root irritation with leg symptoms and, if so, whether the pain is predominantly in the back or leg, and above or below the knee. However, rather than getting bogged down with 20 years of symptoms, asking the patient 'Where is the worst pain today?' will establish whether the pain is predominantly in the mid back, low back, buttock, lateral thigh or radiating below the knee. Also, ask the patient about impulse pain. Pain radiating below the knee, particularly if there is any numbness, tingling or weakness in the leg is an expression of nerve root irritation.

Figure 4.1 shows the main categories of back pain. Finally, examination will show whether the localized pain can be recreated by pressure over specific sites. For individuals who do not fit the above criteria, further investigations may be necessary.

## 4.5 Given the limited time in general practice, what is the best way to examine this sort of case?

A history will help determine whether the symptoms are predominantly in the back or leg (Fig. 4.1) and the examination of the lower limbs followed by back will focus attention on the relevant pathology.

For individuals in whom back pain is the main concern, the lower limbs can be ignored and local palpation (which takes under a minute) will determine the site of relevant pathology (see next question).

Once a mechanical or ligamentous condition is suspected, the history and examination may then reveal the following:

- Back pain only, without radiation, impulse pain, tingling or spasm
- Back pain with spasm
- Back pain with referral to the knee
- Back pain with referral to the foot, in one or both legs, with or without tingling.

## Back pain only

## 4.6 What if the pain is predominantly in the low back with no radiation down the leg and no impulse pain?

This is the commonest problem. Depending on the site, there would be ligamentous pathology at the right or left iliolumbar ligament insertion or that of the interspinous ligaments at the site shown (Fig. 4.2).

On examination you should try to recreate the pain by pressure or have the patient recreate it by a certain movement such as bending forward or sideways. Normally, movement would be painful but not result in spasm. Muscle spasm usually suggests a deeper pathology such as facetal joint dysfunction (rare) or nerve root irritation, secondary to a disc (rare). Next, with the patient lying prone you should put pressure over the interspinous ligaments between L2 and 3, 3 and 4, 4 and 5 and L5 and S1. The

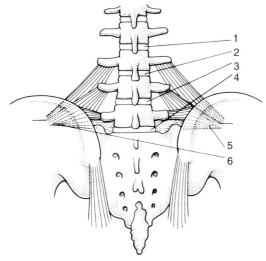

**Fig. 4.2** Local sites of ligamentous pathology, and the relative order of frequency. 1 = interspinous ligament between L2 + L3, 2 = interspinous ligament between L3 +L4; 3 = interspinous ligament between L4 + L5; 4 = interspinous ligament between L5 + S1; 5 = right iliolumbar ligament insertion into superior iliac spine; 6 = left iliolumbar ligament insertion into superior iliac spine. The local sites of tenderness in order of frequency are 3 > 4 > 5 = 6 > 2 > 1.

iliolumbar ligament insertion on the right or left should be examined, and this simple manoeuvre would usually produce the site of pathology (Fig. 4.2). Patients will clearly report the site at which pressure creates the pain.

### 4.7  Is it possible to pinpoint sacroiliac joint pain?

No. The sacroiliac joints are particularly deep and although back pain 'specialists' have claimed that sacroiliac joint pain is recognizable, this is unlikely. Sacroiliitis itself, as part of the inflammatory disease AS may be recognizable but so-called sacroiliac 'strain' probably does not exist. Various manoeuvres have been carried out which purport to 'stress' the sacroiliac joints, resulting in recrudescence of the pain but again this would appear to be improbable. I think that most patients who are said to have pain emanating from the sacroiliac joint in fact have the more superficial iliolumbar ligament insertional tendinitis (Fig. 4.2). The tender site is somewhat lateral to the deep-seated sacroiliac joints and, of course, more superficial.

In fact, in patients with clearly defined sacroiliac disease such as the exceptionally rare septic sacroiliac joint, the pain is widespread and diffuse, radiating into the low back, buttock and thigh rather than being localized to one point.

### 4.8  Is it possible to pinpoint muscle tears?

Partial muscle tears, or ligamentous tears are a cause of acute onset severe back pain and may be associated with muscle spasm. Typically, the patient may report sudden onset of pain after minimal trauma. For example, simply bending down to open a lower drawer, or leaning over a car seat to lift out a briefcase, may cause a stabbing or sudden 'burning' pain in the back. However, these sorts of presentation usually relate to superficial problems rather than to more sinister discogenic disease.

Very local tenderness on palpation will suggest that a partial tear is the cause of the symptoms. However, muscle spasm is more likely to be due to a deep-seated lesion of the facetal joint or nerve root irritation.

### 4.9  How can ligamentous inadequacy be recognized?

Specifically, the onset of pain is rarely sudden and is usually diffuse in nature. The patient will find it difficult to point to one specific location.

The individual is often obese, unfit and perhaps a smoker. The back pain is associated with poor posture and poor musculature, resulting from ligamentous strain or 'inadequacy'. The patient may be more symptomatic early in the morning after a night on a poorly sprung mattress and again will ache during the day when standing.

### 4.10  How should a case of back pain without impulse pain be treated when presenting within the first 2 weeks?

If a patient has back pain without impulse pain the chances that the problem will resolve without any specific management is probably 90% over the next 3 or 4 weeks. You should only become concerned if the trouble has persisted for at least 6 weeks.

Treatment should consist of reassurance, simple analgesics, minimal rest (e.g. 2 days maximum) and advice to continue at work since prolonged rest often causes more rather than fewer long-term problems.

## 4.11  How should these patients be managed when they present later?

If a patient has had low back pain for several weeks without impulse pain they should be treated by local injection if there is a local trigger site. This would typically be at the iliolumbar ligament insertion location or at an interspinous space, most frequently between the 4th and 5th lumbar vertebrae or between L5 and S1. Non-steroidal agents taken orally may help but local treatment for local pathology is best. Swimming is the preferred exercise.

## 4.12  Is chronic ligamentous back pain curable?

Yes. We often see patients who have had back pain for a decade or longer, and in such a situation the good prognosticator is whether the patient can point with one finger to one site of pain. If the patient can localize the pain in this way, a local ligamentous lesion (e.g. at the iliolumbar ligament insertion site or interspinous ligament site in the low back) is likely, and therefore a single local corticosteroid injection at the trigger site may result in a long-term cure.

## 4.13  What lifestyle advice should be given to patients with back pain?

First, try to persuade the patient to stop smoking. There is a good correlation between tobacco and back pain. There are at least three reasons for this. The first is that persistent coughing may be associated with muscle or ligamentous damage and, of course, an underlying painful condition will come to light as the patient coughs. Secondly, the smoker is less likely to be fit and may therefore have weaker musculature and worse posture and is set up for the inevitable vicious cycle. Thirdly, data have suggested that the nicotine in tobacco acts as an antifibrinolitic factor. The effect of this is that microtrauma results in scarring rather than repair and, in turn, the scarring results in more pain.

I would advise the patient to stay fit or to get fit. There is no doubt that good abdominal and spinal musculature will prevent many soft-tissue back problems. The best activity is swimming, which is the natural way to increase particularly the spinal musculature.

Inevitably, excess weight is bad for posture, which, in turn, is bad for the back and so I would recommend that the body weight should return to a 'normal' value.

## 4.14  What exercises should be recommended?

In general, exercises should form an early part of the treatment advice. In the long term, exercises may well prevent a recurrence of the pain. In the short term, exercise may solve the problem.

For the lower back, the patient should carry out lumbar isometric flexion exercises — also known as pelvic tilt exercises. The patient is asked to lie flat on the back on the floor or firm bed. The GP (physiotherapist or spouse/friend) then attempts to insert the hand between the buttock and bed while asking the patient to push down on the hand to prevent the hand from being inserted. While this happens, the normal lumbar lordosis becomes exaggerated and the small of the back lifted off the bed. To counteract this, the therapist inserts the other hand under the small of the back and asks the patient to push down at the same time thus preventing either hand being inserted between the body and the support. This flattens out the normal lumbar curve while tightening the abdominal muscles, paraspinal lumbar muscles and buttock muscles. In this position, the patient counts five slowly and then relaxes completely. The sequence is repeated 10 times thrice daily.

Without doubt the best exercise programme is that of swimming, given that the water buoys the patient and allows remedial exercises for the paralumbar musculature without causing any strain to ligaments or joints. The best activity is crawl or back stroke rather than breast stroke which may cause strain for the hips, knees or shoulders.

## 4.15  When should a corset or cervical collar be considered?

Virtually never. A corset is an anathema to a rheumatologist. We are interested in strengthening the musculature, not the reverse. Unfortunately, too often we see patients who have been in a corset for months or years. We try to extricate them from this in the hope that a good exercise programme will enhance the musculature, resulting in long-term improvement.

Collars are over-used by the patient. There is no reason why a support should not be given for 48 hours but longer than this can result in muscle weakness, deteriorating posture and increasing symptoms. The one exception is the patient with a damaged cervical spine either from trauma or from rheumatoid disease. Such an individual would benefit from a support, at least while travelling, if the spinal cord is at risk from an unstable cervical spine (see Chapter 3).

Inevitably, a long-term hard collar results in no movement and therefore more wasting and so, even in a patient with spinal damage, attempts must be made to support the spine with neuro-surgical intervention where possible.

### 4.16 What is the place of simple analgesics in the treatment of back pain?

Simple analgesics may be appropriate during the acute painful stage. The main benefit is to allow the patient to carry out remedial exercises. Simple analgesics are always safer than NSAIDs and should be tried as the first line of therapy. Only when the analgesics are inadequate should the non-steroidal agents be given. In conjunction with simple analgesics I would advise the patient about ice packs or possibly a hot-water bottle. In general, some 80% of individuals prefer ice, while 20% get benefit from heat. The advantage of an ice pack is that it can be placed locally at the site of maximum pain and may well break the vicious cycle in a way that an analgesic or non-steroidal agent will fail to do.

### 4.17 What is the role of local corticosteroid injection?

In general, local pathology should be treated with local treatment. Clearly, such an approach avoids the systemic effect of drugs and the relative inefficacy that may be expected from a non-steroidal or analgesic agent at a site distant from the mouth and stomach. Local pathology may well respond to local corticosteroid infiltration. In general, a long-acting agent is used together with local anaesthetic. Favoured injection sites include the greater trochanteric bursa, subperiostally at the iliolumbar ligament insertion, the interspinous ligaments particularly between L3 and 4, the L4 and 5 and the L5 and S1 and perhaps at the interspace between C5 and C6 and C6 and C7 in the neck. Other trigger sites around muscle insertion into the scapulae may be dealt with in a similar manner. In general, if symptoms have been persistent for more than 6 weeks I would inject. If multiple trigger sites are present, a trial of a non-steroidal agent would be appropriate.

## Pain radiating down the leg

### 4.18   What if the pain radiates to the knee?

Pain in the lateral thigh not radiating below the knee suggests a greater trochanteric bursitis (Chapter 6). Hip pain, by contrast, is felt medially in the groin and upper thigh; it can also radiate to the knee, sometimes causing confusion. A careful examination will define the precise location of pathology.

Rarely a patient presents with so-called 'meralgia paraesthetica'. This relates to pressure on the lateral cutaneous nerve of the thigh as it passes by the anterior iliac spine. Pressure at this site will recreate the feeling of pain, tingling and numbness in the lateral thigh. The typical situation is where there is entrapment of the lateral cutaneous nerve in an individual who has recently increased in weight but still wears the same old, now tight trousers and pressure from the trouser or belt causes damage to the underlying nerve.

## Back pain with nerve involvement

### 4.19   What if the pain radiates down one or both legs?

Discomfort predominantly in the anterior compartment suggests L3/4 nerve root irritation, and in the lateral compartment suggests L4/5 involvement; pain down the back of the leg is suggestive of L5/S1.

In the example in Table 4.3, the left leg elevation results in pain at 50 degrees compared with the normal 80 degrees on the right and when the left foot is flicked back (sciatic nerve stretch) the patient complains of pain. However, it is not too severe because, as noted next, there is no increased pain down the contralateral normal leg. Sensation (simply running the fingers down both shins anteriorly, laterally and medially) is normal but the left foot is somewhat weaker when the foot is twisted out compared with the normal right side. Knee reflexes, as expected, are normal but the ankle jerk is decreased. This tells us that the

**Table 4.3** Main findings on examination in the case of L5/S1 nerve route irritation (see text)

|  | Right | Left |
|---|---|---|
| Straight leg raising | 80 | 50 |
| Sciatic nerve stretch | – | + |
| Crossed sciatic nerve stretch | – | – |
| Sensation | Yes | Yes |
| Power | Yes | Decreased plantar flexion of foot |
| Reflexes |  |  |
| Knee | ++ | ++ |
| Ankle | + | – |

left L5/S1 nerve root is irritated and appropriate management can then be initiated. If, by contrast, there are no differences in the two sides then it is certain that there is no sinister pathology and the attention can be focused on the spine with the likelihood of one of the tender sites demonstrated in Figure 4.2 being found. In general, if this is the situation (i.e. predominant back pain with some leg pain radiation but no leg neurological findings) treatment directed towards the back will solve the problem.

## 4.20  What is the significance of impulse pain?

If pain radiates down the leg on coughing or sneezing it may be assumed that a nerve route is entrapped by an osteophyte or disc. The distribution of the pain helps locate the site of nerve root irritation (e.g. L4/5 or L5/S1).

## 4.21  Can disc tears cause back pain with nerve involvement?

Disc tears are an unusual cause of back pain. Most patients who are said to have a 'prolapsed disc' or 'slipped disc' have neither, and such a diagnostic label should be avoided unless there is clear evidence of sudden-onset nerve root irritation with pain clearly radiating down the L4/5 or L5/S1 distribution, often with marked physical findings and almost always impulse pain. In such individuals, a CT scan or MRI study will confirm disc prolapse through the torn annulus. A straight radiograph of the spine may show disc narrowing but this is irrelevant in terms of pathology — most individuals with disc space alteration visualized on plain film are symptom-free.

## 4.22 Can facet joint dysfunction be responsible for back symptoms?

Facet joint disease as a cause of back pain is most unusual. Unfortunately, the radiological report often suggests that there is 'degenerative change' of the facetal joint and it is easy to assume that this is the cause of the patient's symptoms.

Facet joint involvement as a cause of back pain is often acute and produces pain on lateral rotation and lateral flexion. The injury may result from picking up a heavy weight in an awkward position or simply leaning over and dragging a case out of a car. The pain is often severe and can cause radiation in the distribution of one of the lower lumbar or first sacral nerve roots. The nerve supply to the facetal joint comes from the corresponding nerve root. Frequently there is marked muscle spasm on lateral flexion. A clinical suspicion may suffice in recognizing facetal joint disease.

## 4.23 How should back pain with radiation to one or both legs be treated when presenting within the first 2 weeks?

If the pain radiates only to the knees you need not be too concerned. However, if it reaches the foot there is clearly nerve root irritation, and if there is evidence of a neurodeficit (reduction in power or sensation) then an epidural injection should be considered sooner rather than later. An injection with 40 mg triamcinolone hexacetonide plus sterile saline (10 ml) should be given via the L3/4 epidural space. However, if seen during the first 2 weeks, the problem may well resolve after a period of 48 hours' bed rest.

## 4.24 What if the pain persists for more than 6 weeks?

For those with pain that persists for longer than 6 weeks, an epidural injection should be the first step in the management programme.

If there is impulse pain then an epidural injection given on a day-case basis is usually indicated. Some of these patients respond, however, to deep infiltration in the interspinous space without the need for an epidural. If a day-case epidural does not work it may be worthwhile admitting the patient for 3 or 4 days to institute appropriate therapy with physio- and hydrotherapy perhaps together with an additional epidural. If the patient is still symptomatic with progressive symptoms and an increasing neurodeficit then an MRI or CT scan is indicated with a view to neurosurgical intervention. Alternatively, a caudal-route epidural may be performed on an outpatient basis.

### 4.25 Does the presence of tingling affect management?

Dysaesthesia (tingling) is of less significance than impulse pain and would not make a great deal of difference to the management, although the prognosis is likely to be less good with tingling than without. Similarly, patients with impulse pain and evidence of a neurodeficit (e.g. loss of ankle jerk, loss of power or sensation) have a worse prognosis.

If a patient has had persistent dysaesthesia for over 6 weeks then an epidural injection would be appropriate with management, as discussed for those with impulse pain.

### 4.26  In general, what is the role of epidural injections in the treatment of back pain with nerve involvement?

There are two forms of epidural that are given frequently. The first is the so called lumbar-root epidural where 80 mg of methyl prednisolone or 40 mg of triamcinolone hexacetonide and 10 ml of sterile saline are injected into the epidural space between the third and fourth lumbar vertebrae. The procedure is usually carried out as a day case and may be performed at the bedside or in theatre. The procedure is comparable to a lumbar-spinal tap in terms of requirement for sterility. There have been few studies confirming its efficacy but there is a consensus that epidurals have a major role.

During recent years, a second form of epidural has become popular: that of the caudal approach whereby the same material is infiltrated via the sacral sulcus some several centimetres below the former site. For the latter, the patient is in the prone position rather than the lateral position favoured for the lumbar approach. Many rheumatologists carry out the caudal epidural on an outpatient basis. There have not been adequate studies comparing the caudal and the lumbar routes.

I tend to favour the lumbar approach if only because, in my

personal experience, several patients who had failed to respond to a caudal injection (in my hands) have fared well with the lumbar approach. However, as inpatient facilities (even on a day-case basis) become less available, more caudal injections will no doubt be performed. The precise mixture is variable — some including a local anaesthetic, while others favour saline alone, sometimes in a bigger volume than the 10 ml mentioned above (see also Chapter 11.) Recently, methyl prednisolone has been (perhaps erroneously) linked with arachnoiditis and therefore I tend to favour the use of triamenolone.

REFERRAL

### 4.27 What is the place of lumbar traction?

I favour neither outpatient nor inpatient lumbar traction. There are few data supporting traction *per se*. Although the term 'traction' suggests that two vertebrae are actually distracted, one from the other, allowing the disc space to enlarge and the pressure on the nerve to be relieved, there is little evidence that this actually happens given that the equipment would have to be much more sophisticated than that usually available in our hospitals. However, if a patient is attached (and therefore motionless) to even poor equipment, enforced bed rest may have a role to play.

### 4.28 When should referral be considered in the treatment of back pain?

A patient should be referred when either the GP or the patient feels that he or she would benefit from a second opinion. Clearly, we do not live in an ideal world and there may well be a long delay in having the patient seen by the specialist of the GP's choice. However, I would consider that there is never an inappropriate referral. The motivation behind the GP's referral may be that additional advice is required or it may be that the GP needs the consultant to support his or her approach to the problem. Alternatively, if the patient feels dissatisfied then it is often a sensible approach to refer the patient and defuse any potentially difficult situations.

### 4.29  To whom should the patient with back pain be referred?

This question is difficult to answer given the variation in cover in different parts of the country. In general, orthopaedic surgeons are trained to operate on joints and fractures and have relatively little experience or interest in backs. If a back requires surgery then, if an orthopaedic surgeon with a special interest in backs is not available, referral to a neurosurgeon is appropriate. In general, I would rather have a neurosurgeon operate in and around the nerve roots.

For most patients, the pathology relates to muscle or ligament insertion into bone, to posture, inflammatory change in bursae or inflammatory disease of the spine (AS). For such individuals referral to the rheumatologist is appropriate. Moreover, rheumatologists effectively specialize in pain and all related pain conditions and should be the first port of call for the patient with back pain.

The situation regarding referral to a physiotherapist depends again on geographic location. Some departments have an open-access policy, whereas others require a referral via a rheumatologist. I think it very important for GPs to understand precisely what physiotherapists are good at and in what situations they are less likely to help. This naturally depends on the individual physiotherapist. Some are superbly trained in the diagnosis and management of spinal problems and will help in terms of both assessment and advice regarding long-term management. They are obviously well equipped to define the appropriate exercise and postural programme for the patient. In addition, physiotherapists frequently assess a patient on one occasion and realize that a further half dozen visits would be unlikely to help. Clearly a two-way discussion is necessary to plan appropriate therapy for a specific individual.

### 4.30  What is your opinion on the role of chiropractic and osteopathy?

Patients very frequently have been to a chiropractitioner or osteopath before reaching my clinic. Clearly, I often see their failures. However, I realize it is easy to have a biased opinion of one's alternative practitioner colleagues. As with GPs or rheumatologists, there are good and bad osteopaths. On many occasions I have had exceptionally good relationships with the good ones! Sometimes we see an osteopath refer a patient to a rheumatologist having appreciated that a sinister underlying pathology may be the cause of the persistent problems. Indeed, I have seen osteogenic sarcomas, fibromyosarcoma and myeloma referred from an osteopath. In summary, the good ones are very good.

One concern regarding these alternative practitioners is the expense. Many treatments rely on a series of visits, all adding to time and financial outlay. There are several very positive points that can be made about osteopaths and chiropractitioners. For example, both tend to specialize in back pain and therefore have amassed a great deal of experience over the years, whereas many GPs have relatively little interest and enthusiasm for managing spinal symptoms. The osteopath's enthusiasm and optimism is also an excellent part of the treatment programme; phenomena that patients may not sense from their own GP. Thirdly, the osteopath has time to listen to the patient and to examine them closely whereas we may be in less of a position to provide the patient with this degree of thoroughness. Fourthly, the success rate of osteopaths and chiropractitioners is often impressive and many of us cannot claim this degree of benefit for our patients. Finally, in my experience, immobile parts of the spine can be readily mobilized by chiropractitioners and osteopaths, saving the patient from many visits to a physiotherapist.

In the ideal situation, the GP, osteopath, physiotherapist and rheumatologist all know the strengths of each other and the patients can be directed appropriately.

### 4.31 What advice should GPs give their patients concerning aids that are available?

The important thing to stress to the patient is that the approach to back pain must be a commonsense one. For example, it is too easy for patients to spend a great deal of money on orthopaedic back pain mattresses when a simple firm mattress will suffice. Secondly, there are a variety of chairs on the market that are expensive and supposedly designed for the back pain sufferer. Again, any sensible chair that gives support is ideal. Although not specifically relating to back pain, there are innumerable diets that are recommended for arthritis and back pain sufferers. Clearly, if any one diet was really better than any of the others, then only one would suffice. We must prevent our patients from spending unnecessary funds on unnecessary unproven treatments.

# 5. Problems of the shoulder and upper limb

Patients frequently present with shoulder pain and the GP must decide if this relates to pain radiating from the neck or whether the joint itself is at fault. Occasionally, it is not the joint but the muscles that are the source of symptoms and conditions such as polymyalgia rheumatica (PMR) should be considered in those with bilateral 'shoulder disease' who predominantly have muscle symptoms and signs rather than clear evidence of joint pathology (i.e. limited active movement, normal passive movement). Radiological evaluation of the shoulder is almost always unhelpful and attention must focus on the history and examination to help with the diagnosis.

For most patients who present with elbow pain the site of pathology is likely to be the lateral epicondyle (tennis elbow) or the medial epicondyle (golfer's elbow) rather than the ulnohumeral joint itself. Pain in and around the wrist typically relates to the base of the thumb and it is the carpometacarpal joint that causes so much 'wrist problem'. The second most frequent wrist symptom is that of medial nerve entrapment while primary disorders of the wrist itself are very infrequent. Degenerative arthropathy affecting the small joints of the hand is common and it takes a careful history and physical examination to provide the physician with a clear diagnosis and treatment plan.

## THE SHOULDER

### 5.1 What shoulder problems is the GP likely to see?

Dislocations will usually present to the accident and emergency department. For every 100 shoulder problems, 97 are capsulitis-related (frozen shoulder, see Q5.6), probably due to a small bleed into the joint (even one drop of blood is an irritant and causes low grade synovitis/capsulitis) resulting in decreased mobility with pain on movement.

For non-joint problems, tendinitis *per se* can also cause a problem — and lesions include those of bicipital or infraspinatus or supraspinatus tendinitis.

Other conditions include calcium hydroxyapatite deposition, calcium pyrophosphate deposition, and one or two other crystal-related problems that can cause an acute and sometimes very painful inflammatory arthritis of the shoulder. Women in their 70s and 80s are especially affected.

Rarely, a synovial cyst may occur, which can dissect down into the anterior chest or posteriorly towards the scapula. PMR and fibromyalgia may also present as a painful shoulder (see later).

## 5.2  What about arthritic conditions of the shoulder?

Primary osteoarthrosis of the shoulder is extraordinarily unusual. However, since osteoarthritis is an end-stage joint failure, any form of shoulder disease can finally result in a degenerative arthropathy supra-added on the primary insult. For example, severe RA with shoulder destruction can be complicated at a later stage by OA as can osteonecrosis of the head of the humerus, old trauma or indeed any other entity.

## 5.3  What is the role of the radiograph in diagnosis?

Almost whatever is seen on the radiograph is of little help with management. Unless you believe that the result of the radiographic examination will alter your approach to treatment it should not be performed. Very rarely a lung tumour (Pancoast tumour) at the apex of the lung can infiltrate the axillary nerve, giving pain, but this may be only once in every 100 000 painful shoulders. In such a situation, a chest radiograph would be more appropriate than a shoulder radiograph.

## 5.4  How should I examine a patient who presents with a painful shoulder?

The first decision that the practitioner has to make is whether the pain is coming from the shoulder or the neck. The best approach is to go straight to the neck and assess its mobility: right to left rotation, right and left lateral flexion; if that fails to recreate the pain, try putting pressure on the top of the head and push down to see if there is any pain radiation from the neck to the shoulder. If the pain is recreated, consider a cervical spine pathology (see Chapter 3).

If the neck is not involved, then take the arm and put it passively through a range of movement to see if such a manoeuvre will recreate the pain. Also, look at mobility, in terms of how high up the back they can put their thumb with extension, internal rotation and adduction. For example, does a woman have sufficient mobility to do up her bra at the back? If the mobility is limited in all directions with pain on the extremes, then a capsulitis exists. There may also be evidence of supraspinatus or infraspinatus muscle wasting — particularly when the problem has persisted for several weeks or months.

### 5.5  How does the duration of symptoms affect the decision to treat?

In general, if symptoms have persisted for more than 4–6 weeks then treatment will be necessary. Often, if it is less than 6 weeks, the odds are that the condition will improve on its own. Obviously there are exceptions. If somebody is going to lose his or her job or is self-employed and has had a bad shoulder for only a week, it may be necessary to treat it immediately. For somebody else you might wait a little longer.

Much of what is seen in general practice is self-limiting and it makes no sense to spend a lot of time and energy writing prescriptions, injecting joints or getting investigations if the condition is only going to be present for days rather than weeks.

### 5.6  What is the differential diagnosis between capsulitis and subacromial bursitis, and how are these conditions managed?

Capsulitis (frozen shoulder) and subacromial bursitis both present with pain and decreased mobility in all directions. Subacromial bursitis (impingement problems) usually presents with a painful arc, weak rotator cuff muscles and sometimes a positive impingement sign — pain on internal rotation and flexion of the humerus to 90 degrees. The problem may arise from rotator cuff strain or, in the older age group, primary impingement of the subacromial tissues. These patients respond to rotator cuff strengthening but resistant cases may require a corticosteroid and local anaesthetic injection into the subacromial space. Immediate relief of the symptoms and signs with the effect of the local anaesthetic confirms the diagnosis. Cuff-strengthening exercises (Q5.7) should be continued to ensure no recurrence.

It is difficult or even impossible to define the differences between a 'subacromial bursitis' and capsulitis of the shoulder. Indeed, therapy is the same, with early corticosteroid injection into the glenohumeral joint, which may be helpful in reducing symptoms during the natural recovery process. Personally, I tend to inject *both* the subacromial space and glenohumeral joint given that differentiating the two sites in terms of primary pathology may be difficult.

### 5.7 What are the main shoulder-strengthening exercises?

Specifically, strengthening exercises begin by increasing the power of the deltoid and the supraspinatus and the infraspinatus muscles. These start to waste within days of the onset of shoulder pain; a hollow is often visible at the top of the shoulder and the bony contours can be felt more easily on the painful side than on the contralateral side. For the first exercise, the patient stands facing a mirror and elevates the arm to 90 degrees (if it can be done without pain) or only to 20 degrees if that is what is possible. Ask them to slowly raise and lower their arm again and to try to do that 10 times, morning and evening. Over successive days, the exertion should increase as the pain decreases. In addition, ask them to go up to their limit where they begin to develop pain then turn the palm anteriorly (facing the mirror), and to go backwards, extending the arm perhaps by 10 or 15 degrees, again repeating this 10 times. As they improve they should be able to get it up to 90 degrees and to do the extension at a 90-degree angle, first without weights and then with a 1lb weight (0.5 kg; a large potato or a can of food) and repeat the procedure with a weight increasing to 2–3lbs.

### 5.8 What are the main tendinitis problems and how should they be treated?

Capsulitis of the shoulder can be associated with supraspinatus or bicipital or infraspinatus tendinitis; occasionally, however, these entities may be seen as separate phenomena.

With supraspinatus tendinitis, pain is found on abduction of the arm in the neutral position (painful arc). Treatment is directed towards the tender site in the tendon sheath, with an appropriately positioned steroid injection. However, my own approach is usually to inject the glenohumeral joint directly and assume that the medication will trickle down the tendon sheath, remembering that the sheath is intimately connected to the capsule.

With lone infraspinatus tendinitis, pain is recreated on external rotation of the shoulder, sometimes against pressure. Occasionally a patient may present with pain only on flexion of the arm with tenderness over the bicipital tendon sheath. For such an individual, with infraspinatus or bicipital tendon problems, infiltration around the respective specific tendon sheath is needed.

However, although the treatment of choice is a well-placed corticosteroid infiltration in the tendon sheath rather than in the tendon itself, the tendon can rupture when this is injected directly. By contrast, appropriately performed intra-articular steroid injections are virtually always safe.

### 5.9  What is calcific tendinitis and how is it managed?

Acute calcific tendinitis, or pericapsulitis, associated with calcium hydroxyapatite crystals, may occur, particularly around the shoulder. This can be an excruciatingly painful disorder requiring opiates over the first couple of days while the problem settles. Intralesional corticosteroid may help, though sometimes even this powerful drug is disappointing in such a situation.

Fortunately, this condition is usually self-limiting and the problem settles within 34 days. A radiograph may or may not reveal some amorphous calcific material present on the film.

### 5.10  What should be done for a patient with a synovial cyst?

In this situation it is worthwhile inserting a needle into the glenohumeral joint and draining the fluid, which comes off quite easily; this is often blood-stained and pretty mucky, and just removing the fluid can help, prior to injecting corticosteroids. Clearly, if the problem persists, then referral to a rheumatologist would be appropriate.

### 5.11  What are your reasons for advocating steroid injection of joints and tendon sheaths?

The goal has to be local therapy for a local problem. The alternatives to corticosteroid injections are: either (1) waiting to see if it resolves spontaneously; (2) giving a non-steroidal anti-inflammatory drug (NSAID) with inevitable cost and potential toxicity; (3) referring the patient to physiotherapy, which may not be particularly useful for the shoulder; (4) referring the patient, for example, to a rheumatologist and hoping that before the patient is seen before the problem will have resolved on its own. Most of the alternatives to early injection are expensive in terms of 'time and energy' or money. Having said that, it is reasonable to try a *short* course of an NSAID (e.g. 10–14 days) since this may break the pain cycle.

### 5.12  Can the GP manage to treat patients with local steroid injection within the busy practice setting?

That very much depends on the format of the practice. For the GP with the experience and interest in setting up an injection session, the patient can be asked to return in 3–4 days when everything is ready, sterile, and the injection material is out. Up to 10 patients can be treated in an hour this way. Obviously, if there is an urgent problem, it will have to be sorted out immediately, and I think there is no easy answer to that. The patient will have to undress, which takes time, particularly if they have reduced mobility. The injections must be performed appropriately. This may create a backlog of patients. For this reason, a GP may find it impossible to take on injection treatment, and patients may have to be referred because of the pressure of work.

### 5.13  What happens when, after treatment, the patient comes back in a month and says, 'Doctor, I'm no better'?

Even if the injection is just right, the success rate is perhaps only 90% if the symptoms have been present for some 3 months. This falls to about 70% if symptoms have been present for 6 months or more. My approach would be to reinject the glenohumeral joint with a larger volume of lignocaine and try to break down any residual adhesions with just a low-dose corticosteroid. Where symptoms persist, you would then have to decide whether to order any investigations. Such a patient attending my clinic would almost certainly receive a suprascapular nerve block with bupivacaine (approximately 10 ml of 0.5% solution). This may well succeed where intra-articular steroid injections have failed.

## POLYMYALGIA AND FIBROMYALGIA

When a patient presents with bilateral shoulder disease, consider a systemic problem such as PMR. This inflammatory condition can present with pain in all the limb girdles or rarely with upper limb symptoms alone.

### 5.14 Can polymyalgia and fibromyalgia be mistaken for capsulitis?

A good point. PMR is always thought of as being a symmetrical disease affecting both shoulder and thigh areas but certainly it can sometimes affect one side first. Probably all of us have been caught out thinking we were dealing with a localized shoulder capsulitis only to find the patient returns at a later stage with the contralateral shoulder involved as well.

Likewise, although a patient with fibromyalgia usually presents with pain 'all over', a more localized problem, with one or both shoulders involved, for example, may be the presenting situation.

### 5.15 How should patients who are suspected of having either PMR or fibromyalgia be examined and investigated?

Without any doubt, the history is of greatest importance followed by the examination. Nevertheless, there will still be the occasional individual where it remains unclear whether one is dealing with non-specific fibromyalgia or PMR. In such an individual an ESR or plasma viscosity will be of great help in ruling out one or confirming the other. However, there are always exceptions and perhaps some 5% of individuals with PMR have a normal ESR. Occasionally one is forced into a trial of corticosteroid. The answer becomes apparent within 24 hours. If a patient is given 30 mg of prednisolone in the morning and has not improved by night or, at the latest, the following morning then the diagnosis is not PMR and one must think again. This steroid trial can be initiated by the GP.

The patient with fibromyalgia will have several painful trigger sites, often a rather long, insidious history, the presence, perhaps, of irritable bowel syndrome and other so-called functional difficulties. Examination will reveal no evidence of arthritis *per se* and the patient often finds it difficult to localize the trouble precisely. However, the worst sites tend to be around the scapula and perinuchal musculature.

One of the major steps in the examination of patients with possible PMR consists of asking the patient to stand, unassisted from a sitting position. In order to do this I tell the patient to fold the arms and to stand up. If the manoeuvre is carried out simply and without difficulty then PMR is unlikely to be the diagnosis. In addition, the patient with PMR is unlikely to be able to clap above the head and behind the buttocks without inducing pain. This is often perceived by the patient to relate to 'shoulder arthritis' but, on examination with passive movement, it becomes clear that the shoulders themselves move well without pain. Interestingly, the patient frequently thinks that the disease relates to the joints (e.g. hip and shoulders) whereas it is the musculature in juxtaposition to these joints that bears the brunt of the disease.

The important features of fibromyalgia and PMR are compared in Table 5.1.

**Table 5.1** Comparison of the main features of fibromyalgia and PMR

|  | Fibromyalgia | PMR |
|---|---|---|
| Age (years) | 20–90 | >60 |
| Sex ratio | F > M | F = M |
| Onset | Insidious, over weeks/months | Often 'sudden', overnight |
| Symptoms | Vague, malaise, poor sleep, miserable — wakes tired, unhappy, tearful, pain all over, irritable bowel syndrome may be present | Upper and lower limb proximal pain and weakness |
| Examination | Tender 'all over' with multiple trigger sites | Localized tenderness to upper arms and thighs, weak proximal musculature, normal joints |
| Laboratory tests | Normal | ESR ↑ Plasma viscosity ↑ |
| Treatment | Exercise, reassurance, Amitryptyline, injection of trigger sites |  |

## 5.16  What is the management of fibromyalgia?

The patient needs a great deal of explanation and advice about the condition. Without education one can never win. Even with time, energy and therapeutic advice one can still fail to help the patient. With fibromyalgia there is little to offer apart from stressing the need for an entirely new approach to the individual's lifestyle.

It should be explained to the patient what he or she does not have. That is to say, it is *not* rheumatoid disease or another sinister entity. A useful analogy is that the generalized pain of fibromyalgia is like the generalized headache — it can be caused by something nasty like cancer of the brain or meningitis but, almost always, it will be a non-threatening cause like non-specific tension either in the frontal or occipital muscles (i.e. headache) or all over (e.g. fibromyalgia).

Next, general fitness and the need to exercise more rather than less should be discussed. General advice about obesity, smoking and other problems should be addressed. It may be worthwhile injecting the odd trigger site. If these simple manoeuvres fail, I would add low-dose amitriptyline at 8 pm. It is important to explain to the patient that their sleep pattern can be improved by low-dose amitriptyline. Again, it is necessary to explain exactly how this should be taken. For example, if amitriptyline is taken later than 8 pm there may be early morning drowsiness. If the dose is too high there may be dryness of eyes and mouth. Once the correct dose is reached by careful titration, this should be continued for several weeks before deciding whether or not the agent has been successful. A GP would usually manage such patients, although the intractable patient should be referred to a rheumatologist.

## 5.17  What is the management of PMR?

If you consider that the patient has a component of giant cell or temporal arteritis then high-dose prednisolone with at least 60 mg daily is warranted, taking the dose each morning with breakfast. Within a few days this can be titrated slowly down from 45, 30, 20, 15, 12.5 to 10 mg, arriving at this lower dose after some 2 months. Thereafter the medication would be continued, decreasing by 1 mg or less per month until a dose of approximately 5 mg daily is reached. Then the dose would be decreased further by monthly decrements of perhaps 0.5 mg. Thus, a patient would be told to take 5 mg alternating with 4 mg for a month followed by 4 mg daily for a month and then 4 mg alternating with 3 mg, etc. By so doing, the aim is to be able to get the patient off corticosteroid therapy within 2 or 3 years.

When treating PMR, I would begin with 30 mg each morning, tapering to 10 mg within 2–4 weeks and thereafter slowly taper again, anticipating cessation of drug therapy some 2 years after commencement. For both giant-cell arteritis and PMR the GP can manage the patient, perhaps relying on a single visit to a rheumatologist for confirmation of the diagnosis and general guidance.

### 5.18 What are the main problems or errors in the management of PMR?

There is a tendency for GPs to stop the medication too quickly. This may well relate to pressure from patients and the natural and correct assumption that steroids are toxic. For those individuals who fail to respond to a low dose (say 5 mg per day after gently tapering the dose over 6 months) the addition of low-dose methotrexate or azathioprine may be appropriate. The patient should be warned that at each dose decrement there may be what appears to be a mini flare-up of the disease. However, this is known as a steroid withdrawal pseudo-rheumatism syndrome. This is well known in the pulmonary literature — patients with asthma, for example, having high-dose prednisolone that tapers quickly often have generalized aches for 3 or 4 days. If, however, the symptoms persist, a higher dose may be indicated.

### 5.19 Do you think that PMR should be managed entirely by the GP?

PMR should be a straightforward condition to manage. However, I think there are occasionally misconceptions that result in some patients having less than optimal care and obviously in such situations referral would be beneficial.

Specifically, we see patients who are under-treated with corticosteroids, on the one hand, whereas a few are over-treated. In general, patients will require at least 2 years of corticosteroid therapy; tapering the patient off all therapy within 6–12 months is too soon in most cases. By contrast, if after 12 months the patient cannot get well below 6 or 7 mg then use of a steroid-sparing agent should be considered sooner rather than later in order to avoid some of the steroid complications.

## 5.20 What steroid-sparing agents are appropriate?

In the past, azathioprine was the usual agent in such circumstances but many of us now favour low-dose methotrexate. It may be possible to taper the prednisolone below 7.5 mg with the addition of 5 or 7.5 mg methotrexate once per week by mouth. Once the disease is well controlled we would probably rather continue to taper the prednisolone, feeling that, over all, low-dose methotrexate is safer than medium-dose prednisolone.

## 5.21 What other concerns are there about the use of steroids such as prednisolone — particularly in the long term — in general practice?

The major issue relates to chronobiology — that is to say the timing of when the drug is given. Unfortunately, we still see patients who are given prednisolone in divided doses and this is almost never appropriate. Prednisolone should be given as a single daily dose in the morning, before breakfast since this will have less effect on the diurnal rhythm of the normal cortisol production. Moreover, a patient who is on a single oral dose is more easily titrated than one on divided doses.

The second issue relates to patients who do not have adequate responses to corticosteroids and the dose is increased but where the reason for a lack of response may, in fact, not have been defined adequately. For example, a patient with PMR requiring more than 3–4 mg prednisolone because of bilateral shoulder pain may, in fact, have a coincidental capsulitis of the shoulder. For such an individual, intra-articular corticosteroid may resolve the shoulder problem and then a more rapid tapering of prednisolone dosage becomes possible. Sometimes, the addition of an NSAID will allow a further reduction in steroid dosage.

Another problem is seen in patients with persisting symptoms who have, in fact, a superimposed fibromyalgia rather than active PMR.

## THE UPPER ARM

### 5.22  What is neuralgic amyotrophy?

This is a relatively rare, perhaps virus-induced disorder that can present with pain, loss of function, weakness and wasting of some of the upper limb muscle groups. Fortunately, the disease is usually self-limiting and there can be return to normal function.

### 5.23  What is the shoulder/hand syndrome?

This is a very important entity that is also referred to as Sudeck's atrophy, reflex algodystrophy, sympathetic dysautonomia, among other labels. In essence, the disease is of unknown aetiology but appears to relate to a painful condition in and around the shoulder, which, in turn, results in a sympathetic dysautonomic phenomenon with increasing pain in the hand, often associated with sweating of the palm, coldness or warmth, loss of function and finally osteoporosis seen on the radiograph. Somewhat earlier than the radiographic change increased uptake may be seen on a radioactive technetium bone scan.

The condition can also follow other painful conditions such as a myocardial infarct, hospitalization with perhaps trauma to the shoulder during the anaesthetic and other possibilities.

### 5.24  How should the shoulder/hand syndrome be treated?

The condition must be treated aggressively. First the patient must receive education and explanation and understand that an aggressive physiotherapy and exercise programme is of paramount importance regardless of the pain. The latter can be suppressed with analgesics or with intra-articular injection into the shoulder or more distally. In addition, for very severe cases, a stellate ganglion block may be required with guanethidine. Additional anti-inflammatory agents, antidepressive drugs and other modalities may be tried but the hallmark of therapy relates to movement. This must include the digits, the wrist, the elbow and the shoulder. Finally, it may be worth frightening the patient with the information that one or two individuals end up with amputations. Perhaps the commonest cause of an algodystrophy in rheumatological practice is a reflex dysautonomia of the hand following minor trauma. The arm may have been placed in plaster and the immobilization triggers the vicious cycle. To avoid this potential catastrophe, casualty officers, orthopaedic trainees and GPs must be told to stress the importance to the patient of continuous hand and shoulder exercises in spite of the plaster. Early referral to a rheumatologist is of paramount importance.

## THE ELBOW

Elbow pain relates to pathology in the elbow joint itself (i.e. the humeroulnar joint), or the radiohumeral joint or — and much more frequently — at the ligamentous insertions medially or laterally. The latter is approximately 10 times more common than the former location. The so-called 'tennis elbow' relates to pathology where the extensor apparatus of the hand arises from the lateral epicondyle. By contrast, on the medial side is the so-called 'golfers' elbow' — pathology at the site of insertion of the flexor apparatus at the medial epicondyle.

More unusual is primary arthropathy of the elbow joint itself — seen typically in patients with generalized inflammatory joint disease (e.g. rheumatoid arthritis — RA, spondylarthritis or psoriatic arthritis).

### 5.25  How do patients with lateral and medial epicondylitis present?

In lateral epicondylitis, the patient feels pain on the outer border of the elbow. This may radiate down towards the wrist and sometimes above the elbow, towards the shoulder. Shaking the patient's hand may cause pain. Typically the patient feels pain on gripping or supinating the hand.

Regarding medial epicondylitis, symptoms are much the same as above but the patient will often point to his or her medial (inner) border of the elbow, again with pain radiating down towards the wrist. The history, however, is much the same given that patients will note pain in and around the elbow on gripping or supinating the hand.

A history can be confusing as both occur together but examination will quickly reveal the precise site of tenderness. When examining the patient it is important to define the precise epicentre given that there are at least half a dozen different pathologies that can result in 'tennis elbow'. For example, synovitis at the radiohumeral joint can cause a similar distribution of pain, while an insertional tendinitis of the orbicularis tendon around the radial head can be the aetiological factor. At the other extreme, an insertional tendinitis of the extensor apparatus is the cause of 'classical' epicondylitis.

### 5.26  What is the treatment of choice for epicondylitis?

Treatment depends on time (leave the patient for 4–6 weeks in case the problem resolves on its own); if it does not resolve, then local steroid infiltration is the treatment of choice. This must be located precisely and the needle must be inserted under the periosteum to avoid subcutaneous atrophy.

One problem with GPs injecting this site is that it is often perceived that the tennis elbow injection is 'easy'. It is worth stressing that intra-articular steroid injections are simple to perform because one knows precisely whether the needle is correctly situated. By contrast, for elbow pain, we see too many patients who have had inappropriate infiltrations in the wrong site and who later present with skin atrophy.

If the problem recurs, I would also teach the patient some strengthening exercises. For example, taking a soft ball and slowly gripping the ball, counting slowly to three and releasing is a helpful way of building up the forearm musculature. Sometimes, a Velcro™ support worn some 8 cm distal to the elbow is helpful. Inappropriate gripping during the day will become apparent to the patient as pressure under the Velcro™ support is noticed.

NSAIDs may decrease symptoms for the first few weeks but persistence in spite of treatment requires injection or referral.

### 5.27  When would a GP refer the patient with persistent epicondylitis on to a rheumatologist or to a surgeon?

The patient should be referred to a rheumatologist for an injection, or if one injection from the GP has failed to cure the patient. In general, one is reluctant to inject more than two or three times before referral to a surgeon. If the patient has not improved following the GP's injection, the patient should be referred on to a rheumatologist. In my experience as a rheumatologist I would refer on to a surgeon perhaps one in every 200 patients who are referred to me. Thus, the orthopaedic surgeon should only very rarely have to deal with surgical intervention in this situation.

In summary, one injection from the GP and one or two from the rheumatologist should suffice. If not, surgery is probably indicated.

## FOREARM, WRIST AND HAND

### 5.28 How helpful is the term 'repetitive strain injury (RSI)'?

This term is undesirable and unhelpful for several reasons. First, it is highly emotive and the meaning changes relating to whether the term is used for medicolegal reasons, as a clinical label or as a sociological problem.

The main problem relating to RSI is that it means one thing to a lawyer and another to the physician. Needless to say, the patient is in the middle and is thoroughly confused (quite appropriately) by the entire story. If it indicates a work-related upper-limb disorder then it has to be unambiguously work-related for obvious reasons. If it indicates 'injury' then equally an injury has to have occurred and this injury must relate to a repeated 'strain'. Given that upper-limb symptoms are extraordinarily common and that there is virtually no relationship between symptoms and working activities, the label 'SRI' should be avoided unless there really is clear evidence of a repetitive strain injury.

For example, there are certain occupational activities whereby inappropriate strain of a highly repetitive nature occurs, without adequate rest and attention to the work situation, and the tenosynovial sheath becomes inflamed, warm, boggy and painful with clear evidence of crepitus. On stopping the work, the symptoms are relieved and on returning to work a similar pathology occurs. This is a very rare circumstance but it exists. In general the famous (or infamous) judge who stated that 'RSI does not occur' was almost right. If he said that it almost never occurs we would be quite happy.

Moreover, every practitioner knows that the term 'tennis elbow' does not mean that the lateral epicondylitis occurred as a result of playing tennis. For this very same reason the term RSI should be avoided unless there is indisputable evidence that this in fact is the just label.

## 5.29  What are the common problems causing wrist pain?

Most patients with wrist pain actually have a degenerative arthropathy of the first carpometacarpal joint, with pain at the base of the thumb rather than in the wrist itself. Tenosynovitis of the tendon sheaths of the extensor tendons as they pass over the wrist and primary synovitis of the wrist itself is also seen. Viral arthropathy, particularly, is often associated with low-grade wrist synovitis but similar changes in patients can be seen with any systemic rheumatological condition such as rheumatoid disease or even PMR.

On the volar side of the wrist, the median nerve can be entrapped, causing a carpal tunnel syndrome (CTS). This is perhaps the most common 'wrist' problem that presents to the rheumatologist, after the first carpometacarpal problems.

There are a variety of miscellaneous conditions that present with wrist and hand pain. Almost certainly these relate to repeated microtrauma and are associated with capsular damage at the wrist or other similar pathology affecting the ligaments and tendons that abound both anteriorly and posteriorly.

The wrist itself rarely, if ever, develops degenerative arthropathy and so most of the wrist conditions relate to soft-tissue pathology.

## 5.30  What is Dequervain's tenosynovitis?

Dequervain's tenosynovitis is an inflammatory disorder of the tendon sheaths around the extensor carpi radialis and the extensor pollicis tendon sheaths. The location of the pain is usually one or two centimetres proximal to the wrist on the radial side. Pain is recreated by extending the thumb and there will be marked tenderness over the extensor tendons. In addition there may be crepitus as the thumb is extended. The treatment of choice is usually corticosteroid injection into the tendon sheath, avoiding the tendon itself. The cause of the problem may be mechanical following an unusual repetitive action or it may be mechanical following a specific action such as lifting a new baby in an awkward position. Alternatively, it can be part of a generalized inflammatory disorder such as RA (Chapter 7).

## 5.31  Can any inflammatory disease cause tendon sheath inflammation?

Yes. However, certain disorders characteristically affect certain tendons and sheaths. For example, gonococcal infection can cause a tenosynovitis anywhere but typically in the forearm such as with Dequervain's tenosynovitis. By contrast, Reiter's syndrome typically affects the Achilles tendon sheath or perineal longus sheath at the lateral side of the ankle (Chapter 6).

## 5.32  What forms of treatment are suitable for tendon sheath inflammation?

There is no doubt that corticosteroid injection gives the most rapid effect in all these conditions. Understandably, many patients will not have the opportunity of being treated by the rheumatologist or other physician knowledgeable in such injection techniques and such an individual may receive an NSAID by mouth, splinting or even a plaster of Paris. However, I doubt if any of these procedures makes a great deal of difference to the natural course. Naturally, many tendon sheath conditions are self-limiting and, regardless of treatment, will improve within 2 or 3 days.

## 5.33  What are causes of median nerve entrapment (CTS)?

CTS (carpal tunnel syndrome or nerve root entrapment) usually has an idiopathic cause. Patients may be born with a narrow canal and any process associated with ageing, degenerative change, repeated trauma or other factor may precipitate the onset of CTS. Naturally, any of the inflammatory synovitides can be associated with nerve root entrapment by way of the increasing bulk of synovial tissue causing pressure at the wrist. Fluid retention from any cause can precipitate the syndrome and the situation frequently occurs during pregnancy, sometimes with fluid retention associated with menstruation in women and also as a result of NSAIDs, which can cause fluid retention. Ironically, we sometimes see patients who present to their GP with CTS and are given an NSAID. Needless to say this can make the matter worse!

Furthermore, any deposition disease can produce symptoms. For example, amyloid (primary or following renal transplantation) may develop into CTS or in fact any of the nerve entrapment syndromes.

### 5.34 What are the symptoms of entrapment neuropathy (CTS)?

The symptoms depend on the location of the nerve. In CTS, the classical teaching is that patients present with dysaesthesiae in the median nerve distribution (i.e. thumb, index finger, middle finger and radial half of the fourth finger). The symptoms most frequently come on at night, waking the patient who responds by shaking the hand to relieve the discomfort. In fact, the median nerve symptoms are usually less well-defined and most patients report pain and tingling in the hand and forearm. Almost certainly there is a marked variation in anatomy and in any case it is difficult for people to localize pain and tingling particularly while asleep! The most important point is that pain can radiate up into the forearm as well as down into the digits. (Tarsal nerve entrapment neuropathy can present with similar symptoms in the distribution of the tarsal nerve while meralgia paraesthetica is associated with numbness and pain in the lateral thigh somewhat reminiscent of a greater trochanteric bursitis.)

### 5.35 How is the diagnosis of entrapment neuropathy made?

Median nerve entrapment or CTS typically presents in women, often in the third or fourth decade but may occur at any age and in both sexes.

The diagnosis is made by close attention to the history followed by an attempt to recreate the symptoms by pressure over the involved nerve. For example, gentle percussion over the median nerve on the volar surface of the wrist recreates the symptoms, as does gentle pressure. Asking the patient to extend the hand backwards, as when adopting the prayer position can also precipitate the symptoms.

It is only by careful examination that the precise location of the problem can be defined. Pressure over the nerve with gentle tapping may produce increasing symptoms in the fingers (Tinel's sign), while, on occasion, none of these manoeuvres can recreate the pain. In such a situation an injection into the carpal tunnel will often cure the problem, demonstrating that the classical textbook teaching often fails to provide all the answers!

### 5.36 How is it possible to tell if the CTS is primary or secondary to another cause?

Usually this becomes obvious on listening to the patient and on examination. Clearly, if a patient has a generalized inflammatory disorder then one need hardly look further for the cause. Sometimes the cause is deceptive, for example, a patient presents with CTS but has occult hypothyroidism — a recognized association. As intimated above, it is always worth asking whether the patient is on an NSAID and also interesting to know whether there is a periodicity following the menstrual cycle. In addition, it is well recognized that a minor degree of entrapment at two sites compounds the problem. For example, an individual may have a narrow carpal tunnel, which, in itself, would not cause problems. However, if there is cervical spondylosis with some nerve root irritation in the neck then the two together may be sufficient to precipitate the clinical syndrome.

### 5.37 Is there a role for nerve conduction studies?

Although the only precise way to confirm the diagnosis of CTS is by nerve conduction studies. I consider this is unreasonable since the procedure is time-consuming and expensive and inevitably the patient will have to wait for the test to be performed and for a physician to get the results. I would therefore always recommend treatment and only if this fails would I suggest further investigations.

### 5.38 What is the treatment of CTS?

From a rheumatological point of view the treatment would always consist of removing the aetiological cause (i.e. stop the NSAID, give a diuretic, treat the hypothyroidism, attempt to suppress the inflammatory joint disease, etc.) in addition to a local injection in an attempt to cure the problem immediately. Only when such a therapeutic approach fails would I consider further investigation. Clearly, if there is already gross loss of function and thenar muscle wasting then an injection is unlikely to help, and urgent referral to a surgeon for carpal tunnel release might be considered. However, I would stress that I think it entirely inappropriate to perform surgery before an injection has been attempted since the success rate with an injection may be 80 or 90% and this improvement can last for years, if not indefinitely. If an injection only helps for a few weeks then again surgical release may be considered. Some surgeons may request nerve conduction studies first but only if the diagnosis is in serious doubt.

### 5.39  A trigger finger is easy to recognize but what causes it?

The commonest cause for a trigger finger (i.e. a stenosing tenosynovitis) is idiopathic. Thus, for no obvious reason, a patient develops a trigger finger. I assume that the actual cause in such situations is mechanical with, for example, repeated hammering, which can traumatize the tendon sheath, which in turn results in a small microbleed causing some tenosynovial inflammation followed by scaring and stenosis. In addition, we frequently see the condition in patients with rheumatoid disease or other inflammatory synovitis that can affect the lining of joints and tendon sheaths equally.

### 5.40  How should a trigger finger be treated?

Without a doubt, the treatment of choice (and indeed almost the only treatment) is a correctly sited injection of corticosteroid into the tendon sheath. I think this is a difficult technique and I would not expect the GP to perform it unless he or she has had direct training from a rheumatologist. The procedure is easily performed given practice but is technically difficult as the tendon itself must not be injected and the procedure can be painful unless performed by an experienced person. The success rate is probably in the region of 99%. In individuals who have repeated episodes but fail to respond to injection, I would refer to a hand surgeon for surgical intervention.

### 5.41  What about more distally? How should a patient who presents with painful fingers be approached?

Almost certainly the commonest cause of a painful finger relates to the distal or proximal interphalangeal joints. Heberden's nodes and Bouchard's nodes are the characteristic changes seen at those two joints respectively. Women are more often affected than men and the condition is often familial. The woman will present with pain, stiffness or swelling of the distal or proximal interphalangeal joints and will be concerned that the disorder is about to spread to more proximal locations. The GP can strongly reassure the patient that this pathology never spreads proximally and the only joints involved would be the distal interphalangeal joints, the proximal interphalangeal joints and interphalangeal joint of the thumb, with involvement of the first metacarpophalangeal joint and the first carpometacarpal joint. The other metacarpophalangeal joints and wrists are spared. There is little correlation between this hand degenerative arthropathy and similar changes in the large weight-bearing joints. With this reassurance the patient is often comforted. In addition, the patient can often be assured that symptoms tend to decrease with time rather than increase. The deformity *per se* may become more evident but there is usually less pain and stiffness over the years. Function remains strikingly normal for the majority of patients.

### 5.42  What is the explanation for swan-neck deformities?

A swan-neck deformity is the result of hyperextension at the proximal interphalangeal joint with resulting hyperflexion at the distal interphalangeal joint. The most common explanation is that of rheumatoid disease whereby the flexor tendon apparatus in the flexor sheath of the digit is damaged at the proximal interphalangeal joint and slips dorsally. The force across the joint now hyperextends that joint rather than flexes it and the resulting fibres to the distant interphalangeal joint now have the effect of hyperflexion at that joint.

# 6. Problems of the hip and lower limb

In the evaluation of lower-limb symptoms, the physician must decide whether pain is radiating from the lower spine down the L4/5 or L5/S1 nerve roots or whether it is hip pain which is radiating to the groin or knee or whether the knee itself is involved as the primary site of the pathology. In general, the history can be confusing but a careful examination will reveal precisely whether one is dealing with nerve root entrapment, primary hip pathology, bursal disease, quadriceps apparatus dysfunction, patellofemoral arthropathy, collateral ligamentous disease at the knee, knee pathology itself or another process.

## THE HIP AND THIGH

### 6.1 What are the common causes of pain around the hip area?

There are many causes of pain in and around the upper thigh that do not actually relate to the hip. Pain in the upper lateral thigh may very rarely relate to hip osteoarthropathy or meralgia paraesthetica (a rare cause) or, as we so commonly see, a greater trochanteric bursitis.

By contrast, sacroiliitis (a manifestation of AS) is diffuse in nature with pain felt in the buttock, low back and sometimes posterior thigh. In such situations, hip mobility will be normal (unless there is hip involvement) without discomfort on the extremes of movement.

However, pain may also radiate from the spine. Facetal joint involvement or even nerve root entrapment can give pain radiating towards the hip and this can confuse the practitioner unless the patient is examined carefully.

Many patients are confused by the location of the pain. In fact, hip pain virtually never presents with upper lateral thigh pain. Hip pain almost always presents with medial groin pain and pain radiating down deeply in the thigh. Occasionally, hip pain can be referred to the knee because of involvement of the obturator nerve.

### 6.2 How can hip pain be differentiated from trochanteric bursa pain?

Differentiating between hip and trochanteric bursa pain is made easier if one listens carefully to the patient. With the latter, rotating on the side at night will recreate the pain whereas hip pain is typically worse on rising after sitting or lying and at least in the earlier stages is less likely to wake the patient.

Pain radiating from the hip is usually associated with decreased mobility of the hip, and pain on the extremes of movement. Internal rotation is often the first to decrease as is extension of the hip with the patient lying prone. As mentioned, hip pain is felt in the groin but there may be radiation towards the knee.

Pain in the lateral thigh and buttock suggests bursitis or even an iliolumbar ligament insertional tendinitis as the cause of the discomfort. Therefore, unless the patient points to the medial thigh/groin area as the site of maximum tenderness, hip involvement is unlikely to be the cause of the pathology.

### 6.3 How should a patient who presents with hip or thigh pain be examined?

Following a careful history, on examination, primary hip pain can be diagnosed if and when movement of the hip recreates the symptoms. With the patient lying supine, gentle rotation of the leg in a medial and lateral direction will recreate the pain. Mobility will be found to be limited. If the hip is flexed and internal or external rotation performed, pain will develop again at the extremes. In a normal individual there should be some 30–45 degrees of external rotation and 20–35 degrees of internal rotation. The latter is usually reduced earlier than the former in patients with degenerative arthropathy. When the condition becomes worse, the patient may lie on the back with the leg held in slight flexion and external rotation.

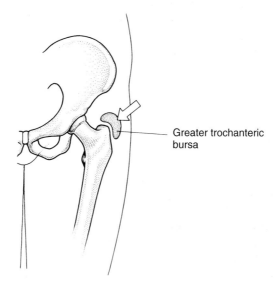

Greater trochanteric
bursa

**Fig. 6.1** Site of maximum tenderness over the greater trochanteric bursa.

If all the above manoeuvres result in no clear recreation of the pain, it may be possible to define hip involvement by lying the patient prone and extending the hip. This should result in some 10 to 20 degrees of extension but this may be less in degenerative arthropathy — again with pain on the extreme. If all these manoeuvres are negative then lying the patient on the side with the leg flexed and internally rotated — thus throwing up the greater trochanter towards the examining hand, may well reveal tenderness over the greater trochanter/bursa in patients with trochanteric bursitis (Fig. 6.1).

### 6.4  How useful is radiological examination of the hip?

Patients are frequently sent for a hip radiograph. Given that most individuals over 50 years of age have some degenerative arthropathy of that joint, the radiological report may suggest that the patient has a definite hip disease. However, history and examination alone may reveal the correct diagnosis without recourse to radiographic examination. This test is appropriate to confirm the diagnosis and for the purpose of planning surgery.

## 6.5  How should hip and thigh trauma injury be managed ?

Tears to the hamstring muscles are common and follow the same rules as calf muscle tears with the emphasis on stretching during recovery. In the young athlete with a lot of bruising around an apparent tear at the origin of either quadriceps or hamstrings, a radiographic examination may be necessary to exclude an avulsion fracture.

Acute adductor strains are common, especially in athletes required to perform a lot of turning and twisting, such as the football mid-fielder. These should be treated as for other muscle problems.

## 6.6  What is the management of hip pain?

Hip involvement itself may respond to simple modalities such as the use of a walking stick on the contralateral side, simple analgesics, a shoe raise on the foreshortened side, advice about posture and remedial strengthening exercises or NSAIDs by mouth. The last of these should only be instigated if other modalities have failed, given the potential toxicity of NSAIDs in the older population.

When all else fails, total hip replacement is inevitable. Given the long delay for many patients on the waiting list for a total hip replacement, a mixture of the above modalities will be tried even in those individuals requiring a total hip replacement. A rheumatologist may well admit the patient as a day case and carry out an intra-articular injection into the hip, which can help for a few months.

## 6.7  What is the management of trochanteric bursitis?

The greater trochanteric bursitis pain is best managed by a local injection. The patient lies on the side that is asymptomatic and the hip is flexed and internally rotated, thrusting the painful trochanteric bursa towards the examining hand. The epicentre is located and injected with one of the long-acting corticosteroid preparations plus lignocaine. This may be performed by the experienced GP or the patient can be referred to a rheumatologist.

## 6.8  What is the management of meralgia paraesthetica?

Patients who present with some lateral thigh numbness and tenderness may have so-called meralgia paraesthetica, which in turn is caused by compression of the lateral cutaneous nerve of the thigh just medial to the anterior iliac crest. This is frequently compressed by a tight belt or trousers, particularly in patients who have gained weight. Again, injection around the compressed nerve is the treatment of choice.

## THE KNEE AND LOWER LEG

Around 80% of the knee support comes not from the structure of the knee but from muscles, in contrast to other joints where the architecture of the joint plays the major role in joint function and support.

### 6.9  What are the common knee conditions presenting to the GP?

There are many problems in and around the knee that can present with `knee' pain and many of these are not age-related.

For those patients who really have degenerative arthritis of the knee joint, the pain may result from synovitis *per se*. If there is inflammation and swelling of the synovium, synovial fluid collects and this, in turn, can produce a popliteal cyst or the patient may have additional extra-articular problems such as the medial and lateral collateral ligament insertional tendinitides or inflammation of the anserine bursa (i.e. the sac between the semimembranosus and semitendinosus ligaments).

In the older population, knee OA is common but it must be stressed that most patients with degenerative arthropathy defined radiologically have no knee symptoms.

One common form of knee pain is that which is worse when the patient walks down rather than up stairs. This is typical of patellofemoral pain. In a young individual we speak of chondromalacia patellae but in older subjects patellofemoral degenerative arthropathy is the usual cause of these symptoms.

### 6.10  What are the important factors to remember when examining the knee?

It is of paramount importance to determine the precise location of the symptoms (pain, swelling, etc.). Only by examination will it be possible to recognize insertional tendinitis of the collateral ligaments, an anserine bursitis, the presence of a popliteal cyst, the presence of weak quadriceps, the nature of the prepatella or infra-patella bursa and, of course, whether there is or is not an effusion. In addition, the hip should always be examined. As mentioned elsewhere, hip disease can present with knee pain, and one must not get caught out by forgetting to ensure that hip mobility is nor-mal and painless.

In summary, in a swollen knee, synovitis and effusion are pre-sent while in the non-swollen knee there must be an explanation for the symptoms such as ligamentous damage of the medial or lateral collateral ligament. (For a comparison of a normal knee, a knee with RA and a knee with OA, see Fig. 6.2.)

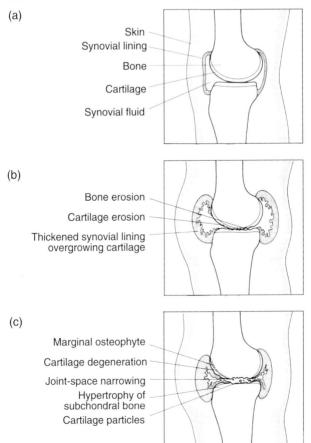

(a)

Skin
Synovial lining
Bone
Cartilage
Synovial fluid

(b)

Bone erosion
Cartilage erosion
Thickened synovial lining overgrowing cartilage

(c)

Marginal osteophyte
Cartilage degeneration
Joint-space narrowing
Hypertrophy of subchondral bone
Cartilage particles

**Fig. 6.2** Schematic diagrams showing the effects of RA and OA compared with a normal knee joint: (a) normal; (b) in rheumatoid arthritis; and (c) in osteoarthritis.

## 6.11  What is the role of further investigations?

If the knee moves well without crepitus or pain on the extremes of movement, no specific investigations are necessary. However, if there appears to be internal damage, then weight-bearing radiographs are appropriate. Most rheumatologists would prefer to see weight-bearing films rather than the more usual supine films that departments of radiology perform unless specifically requested to do otherwise. The reason for weight-bearing films being preferred is that the joint-space narrowing secondary to cartilage loss often only become apparent in the weight-bearing position. Occasionally, films that were taken when the patient was supine appear virtually normal but when the same patient is standing there is clear evidence of medial or lateral compartmental joint space damage.

If there is a suggestion that the problem could be inflammatory in nature, an ESR or plasma viscosity together with a full blood picture and platelet count is helpful. Rheumatoid disease virtually never presents as a single swollen knee and so a rheumatoid factor will almost certainly be negative and when positive, is probably an irrelevant chance finding (remember that 5% of normal individuals are rheumatoid-factor-positive).

## 6.12  What other clinical features should be sought by the GP?

Always look for evidence of systemic disease such as psoriasis or psoriatic nail disease. Psoriatic arthropathy is often asymmetrical and can occur at any age and large joint swelling such as knee arthropathy is not unusual. Close inspection of the nails and skin will give the diagnosis. Even when a cursory glance at the skin is negative, closer inspection of the gluteal cleft, umbilicus or scalp region may reveal a plaque of psoriasis, for example.

## 6.13  When is knee joint aspiration appropriate?

Joint fluid may be aspirated to help with diagnosis. Usually there is little need for such a procedure but rarities include, for example, pigmented villonodular synovitis (PVNS). In such a case, dark blood-stained fluid is the norm.

Fluid should also be analysed from a patient presenting with acute synovitis in whom crystal disease or infection is suspected.

A search for crystals and infective agents would then be mandatory. For patients with chondrocalcinosis on the radiograph (calcium pyrophosphate deposition in the fibro- or hyaline cartilage), synovial fluid analysis for calcium pyrophosphate crystals is appropriate.

In patients with a large effusion there may be compromise of joint function. In such individuals it may be appropriate to drain the fluid, which in turn results in immediate improved function. Some of the knees we see contain 100–200 ml of synovial fluid and removal of this allows improvement of quadriceps action and, of course, results in less pain and improved function. Smaller effusions do not require drainage since the joint will respond well to intra-articular corticosteroid injections.

### 6.14  What are the common sports-related injuries?

With the knee being the most commonly injured joint in sport, the GP will see many injuries early in the natural history. Often the patient will tell of a 'crack' or 'pop' at the time of injury implying significant damage to the knee, anterior cruciate ligament (ACL), collateral ligament injury, torn menisci or other pathology.

### 6.15  How should a GP manage a patient presenting with an acutely painful knee following trauma?

If the knee swells immediately (within 20 to 60 minutes) there has been bleeding into the joint and it is important to make a diagnosis. This usually means arthroscopy and if this service is available acutely, immediate referral is necessary since some of the pathology is correctable in the early stages. The most likely injury is to the anterior cruciate ligament, which is occasionally avulsed from the bone at either end. Unlike the more common mid-substance tear, these avulsions can be reattached.

Collateral ligament injury, more commonly the medial, torn at the upper end on the femoral condyle, is treated in a similar fashion to ankle ligament injury.

Torn menisci are diagnosed mostly from the history — often a twisting injury on a weight-bearing knee with late and persistent swelling and perhaps sharp pains and giving way later. Locking (episodes of loss of full extension) only happen with bucket handle tears, which are rare. The presence then of a continuing effusion, joint line tenderness and perhaps loss of a few degrees of hyperextension may confirm the diagnosis and indicate referral for surgery.

Damage to the outer rim of the meniscus causes bleeding and here the meniscus can sometimes be sutured. Osteochondral fractures present also as haemarthrosis and sometimes need local fixation. If early arthroscopy is not available it is helpful to aspirate the blood, confirming the presence of blood, removing as much as possible and thus reducing discomfort. (Intra-articular corticosteroid injection will lessen the irritant effect of blood, including further synovitis and inflammation.)

Immobilization is only indicated for a severe injury that requires invasive surgery. In general, for most lesser injuries, support and early mobilization reduce recovery time. Concentration on non weight-bearing exercise (cycling and swimming) during healing is useful and, as for the ankle, rehabilitation ensures full range of movement, good muscular support and normal proprioception. Knee exercises tend to concentrate on the quadriceps muscles even though good knee function requires a balance between quadriceps and hamstrings, and after ACL injury the hamstrings are more important.

### 6.16 What if the knee becomes progressively more swollen and painful over several days?

Often, the actual aetiology is less important than the treatment plan. If blood-stained fluid is drawn off from the knee, it clearly suggests a traumatic origin. In this circumstance, if the knee is injected it is likely to improve, and that will be the end of the episode.

Of course there are other more sinister possibilities, such as a cartilage injury, and these will not settle down with any simple treatment modality and within a month or 6 weeks the patient will be back, still with pain (although perhaps no longer any swelling). The important thing to notice here is whether there is any quadriceps wasting. If the quadriceps is still weak and there is still discomfort and it is not obviously swollen, then it should be assumed that there could be a mechanical injury and this would be the sort of case to refer to an orthopaedic surgeon — hopefully one that would be able to consider arthroscopy, sooner rather than later, if necessary.

### 6.17  What if the individual presents with a single painful and somewhat swollen knee, with no other symptoms or signs suggesting a more generalized disease?

An individual may have a swollen knee that persists because the initial inciting event (long since forgotten) may have been a minor traumatic episode with a tiny intra-articular bleed. This results in an inevitable low-grade synovitis since blood is an irritant. Every time the knee begins to settle, the now slightly inflamed synovium rebleeds and the vicious cycle continues. Management therefore, should usually include an intra-articular corticosteroid injection and close attention to the quadriceps apparatus, which needs to be strengthened through exercise.

### 6.18  What are the systemic causes of a swollen knee?

A patient with systemic disease may be young or old (with most being in the third, fourth or fifth decade). The patient should always be questioned about urethritis, mouth ulcers, diarrhoea and other stigmata of Reiter's syndrome/spondylarthritis, given that the commonest cause of an inflammatory swelling of the knee in a young (male) adult would be one of the inflammatory seronegative arthropathies, or reactive arthritis as it is known. For example, occult bowel infection (which may not be occult — there may have been a diarrhoeal episode 2 weeks previously) or a sexually acquired infective episode, such as *Chlamydia* spp. infection or ureaplasma, may result in a reactive response in the knee. Obviously between these two extremes of trauma and a haemorrhagic synovitis on the one hand and a reactive arthropathy in a genetically susceptible individual on the other (precipitated by *Salmonella, Shigella, Yersinia, Campylobacter* spp. in terms of bowel infection, or *Chlamydia* spp. or ureaplasma in terms of sexually acquired infection), there are many other causes of a swollen knee.

### 6.19  When should an infective condition be suspected?

In a patient who is not immunocompromised (on corticosteroids, immunosuppressive therapy, or diabetic), infective mono-arthropathy in the UK is very unusual. Yes, you will find gonococcal arthropathy occasionally but for every 30 patients with a gonococcal swollen knee, 29 will be women, so try to forget that possibility in a male. If, when you draw fluid from the knee, it is cloudy then it must be cultured, which will help the diagnosis. In addition there might well be a story of a urethritis or vaginal discharge but again be prepared for women with gonococcal arthropathy to have minimal or no vaginal symptoms to lead you to that diagnosis. Inevitably, with the increase in HIV positivity and AIDS, the occasional patient presenting with a septic arthropathy and occult AIDS will be seen. In such patients the organism may be unusual.

## 6.20 Clearly local steroid injection is contraindicated in patients with an infected joint. What about local antibiotic injection?

This is a good question. In general, if it is gonococcal disease the gonococcus is exquisitely sensitive to penicillin and oral or, if necessary, intravenous antibiotics are indicated. The knee itself is not irrigated with antibiotics except in very unusual circumstances. Typically, systemic oral, intravenous, or intramuscular antibiotics would be the appropriate route.

## 6.21 In whom would gout be suspected?

In the 20-year-old patient, gout would be extraordinarily unlikely and, in effect, gout is not seen below the age of 45 years. If a young individual has gout, almost always the diagnosis will be self-evident in terms of a very positive family history. They will often already be overweight, hyperlipidaemic, hypertensive and probably abuse alcohol but this again would be a very unusual situation and so it is important not to respond automatically by measuring serum uric acid since this will usually be unhelpful.

## 6.22 What further examination would be necessary if the knee pain is associated with a normal joint?

Regardless of age, we frequently see patients presenting with knee pain who have a normal joint *per se* but evidence of a right or left lateral or medial collateral ligament insertional tendinitis either at the origin (femoral side) or at the insertion (tibia/fibula side). In such individuals, although pain is described as occurring in the knee, it is clear on further discussion that the pain is predominantly medial or lateral and proximal or distal. A brief examination will reveal no joint effusion but marked tenderness at the origin of insertion of one of the collateral ligaments. Again, treatment is directed towards the tender site with subperiosteal steroid injection and attention to the quadriceps apparatus.

Having examined the knee in terms of presence of tender sites or effusion and popliteal cyst, mobility is then assessed. A popliteal cyst is usually associated with pain on forced flexion of the knee. If a patient can flex the knee fully it is very unlikely that there is any major effusion.

### 6.23  What is an anserine bursitis and how is it managed?

Inferomedially to the knee, the semitendinosus tendon passes in close juxtaposition to the semimembranosus tendon and between the two is a bursa known as the anserine bursa. This can become inflamed in any patient with primary knee disease and the diagnosis is made by noticing that the patient is exquisitely tender when the bursal site is pressed. Intrabursal corticosteroid would be the treatment of choice, together with quadriceps exercises.

### 6.24  What is housemaid's knee?

Although every medical student is taught about 'housemaid's knee' this rarely presents in modern medicine. However, we do see a similar problem in individuals who earn their profession on their knees — the most common perhaps being carpet layers. Recurrent trauma to the infrapatella or prepatella bursae results in swelling anterior to the knee and the so-called 'housemaid's knee'. Drainage of the synovial fluid and intrabursal injection will cure the problem.

### 6.25  How should a patient with popliteal or baker's cyst be managed?

A popliteal cyst does not need treatment *per se* in terms of injecting or removing the cyst. By contrast, if we deal with the anterior knee — i.e. by intra-articular injection — this should help the fluid reabsorb and thus allow the popliteal cyst decreases in size. Occasionally the popliteal cyst can rupture as discussed in Q6.26. This typically happens in individuals who have had recent-onset knee swelling because it is the thin synovial lining that bursts. Once the synovial lining and capsule become thickened it is less likely to leak or rupture.

## 6.26 How should a patient who presents with an acutely inflamed, painful calf that can follow rupture of the popliteal cyst be managed?

It is important to consider deep vein thrombosis in this setting but remember that a ruptured popliteal cyst is probably the most likely diagnosis. Such an individual requires early intra-articular corticosteroid injection and should be advised to exercise gently, allowing the anti-inflammatory material to seep down into the calf, reducing the symptoms. Of course, if a deep vein thrombosis is highly suspected on clinical grounds then a venogram would be required to confirm or refute that possibility. Very rarely, a deep vein thrombosis develops as a complication of a ruptured popliteal cyst.

## 6.27 How should calf injury in general be managed?

Partial tears of the calf are common, often with the feeling of being hit on the calf, and the resulting bleeding is a major irritant. Ice packs are again helpful along with elevation and perhaps NSAIDs. After the initial period, it is important to stretch gradually the repairing muscle so that as full healing takes place, it is not shortened by scar tissue, which would make it more at risk from future injury.

## THE ANKLE AND FOOT

## 6.28 What are the most common causes of ankle and foot pain?

I would include the first metatarsophalangeal (MTP) joint, heel pain, ankle pain resulting from medial and lateral ligament dysfunction, general aching related to pes planus (flat foot) and Achilles tendinitis.

Metatarsalgia is the name given to a variety of forefoot problems ranging from common MTP dysfunction to the rare globus tumour, which is usually located between the second and third metatarsal heads.

It is important to remember that the hindfoot moves separately from the mid-foot, which, in turn, moves in different directions from the forefoot and each part must be carefully examined. A final point perhaps is that radiographs are often unhelpful and careful examination is required to elicit the site of pathology.

### 6.29  How should sports injuries resulting in ankle injury be managed?

Clinically, it is often quite difficult to differentiate acute trauma to the ligaments surrounding the ankle from fractures of the fibula or other bones in juxtaposition to the ankle. Soft-tissue injuries are much more common than bony injuries. When there is doubt, a radiograph will be required. The rest of the discussion deals with soft-tissue sports injuries.

In the first 24 hours the application of ice (with the skin suitably protected from freezing) will reduce the bleeding from acute injuries and will give analgesia. Elevation and compression during this time may also help. High doses of NSAIDs (e.g. ibuprofen 2400 mg per day) may also reduce recovery time. For minor ligament strains support in the form of a stirrup strapping will support the ankle and enable early mobilization. Even if it is not possible to weight-bear, it is necessary after the first-aid period to move the joint actively, reducing muscle wasting and helping to relearn the proprioception. Immobilization is only justified when there is severe ligament damage as evidenced by, for example, a positive anterior drawer test: the tibia is stabilized with one hand and the heel cupped in the other. The heel is then pulled at right angles to the tibia. Any movement (in contrast to the other ankle) is abnormal and signifies a major ligament injury.

As the swelling settles it is important that the patient regains a full range of movement of the ankle, full power in the surrounding muscles and a normal proprioception.

### 6.30  What are the likely causes for an ankle strain not recovering?

It is common for patients to complain of weak ankles after a strain. This is due either to an inadequate range of movement, weak controlling muscles (most commonly the peroneal muscles, which support the lateral side of the ankle) or poor proprioception. The last is the most common cause and the use of a wobble board is helpful as an instruction on balancing exercises. It is rare for ligament weakness alone to cause symptoms and full rehabilitation is usually possible with emphasis on the above three elements.

If there is a continuing intra-articular effusion (with fullness, posteriorly, deep to the Achilles tendon) not responding to NSAIDs or physiotherapy, other pathology should be considered such as a non-traumatic cause or damage to the talar dome. The latter is often not evident on the initial radiograph and may need a CT scan for diagnosis.

Finally, blood is an irritant. If symptoms persist, these may relate to a low-grade blood-induced synovitis, which in turn would respond to intra-articular steroid.

### 6.31  What is the approach to a patient who complains of ankle pain?

The history is usually unhelpful because the localization of the pain is poor. Nevertheless, examination readily reveals the site of the pathology. There will be marked tenderness on the medial, or more commonly lateral, side of the foot over the medial and lateral ligaments respectively.

### 6.32  How should these cases be managed?

In general you should ensure that the patient has appropriate supporting footwear and you should have the individual carry out exercises for the intrinsic musculature. Local injections are often very helpful — analogous to the treatment of tennis elbow or knee arthropathy.

### 6.33  What is Achilles tendinitis and how should it be managed?

Achilles tendinitis is a common sports-related condition. The tendon is particularly at risk in repetitive sports and in the older age group when the blood supply to the tendon may be impaired. In the early stages, the inflammation may be restricted to the paratenon and at this stage will respond to electrotherapy from a physiotherapist and perhaps NSAIDs along with gentle stretching.

Since foot biomechanics may contribute to the aetiology, it

may be that temporary use of an appropriate orthosis in the shoe may be effective, reducing the torsional forces on the tendon. If this fails, infiltration of a weak steroid into the area of the tender paratenon alongside the tendon may be effective. The risk of injection into the tendon is small because of the resistance in the tissues to intratendon injection. However, care should be taken and a specialist opinion sought. The tenosynovial sheath, although not real as at other locations in the body, can also be 'inflamed'. Local injections can be potentially dangerous since a misplaced infiltration can result in tendon rupture. Exercise must be directed towards gentle stretching exercises to enhance mobility and the blood supply.

There is a bursa deep to the lower end of the Achilles tendon that is inflamed occasionally. This responds well to steroid injection, which is directed from either side about 5 mm anterior to the tendon immediately above the calcaneum.

### 6.34  What other tendon problems exist?

All the ligaments passing in close juxtaposition to the heel can be associated with a tenosynovitis of the associated tendon sheaths. Careful examination will reveal the precise location of the pain and therefore the pathology.

### 6.35  Is there a pathology in the foot comparable to the carpal tunnel syndrome in the hand?

Yes. The tarsal tunnel syndrome is recognized, although this is much rarer than its equivalent in the hand. Treatment is, however, the same — steroid injection into the tarsal tunnel, relieving pressure on, in this case, the tarsal nerve.

### 6.36  What is plantar fasciitis and how should it be managed?

Plantar fasciitis (painful heel) is common in runners and non-sportsmen and is often associated with biomechanical problems such as overpronation of the foot caused by a varus deformity of the forefoot in relation to the rearfoot. It may be related to poor footwear or exercise. It responds well to steroid injection into the area of the anterior calcaneum and some consider it best to approach this area from the medial aspect of the heel. It may be associated with a heel spur but this does not change the management since such spurs are irrelevant radiological findings — there being no relationship between spurs and symptoms. An orthosis in the shoe may be necessary. Plantar fasciitis can be differentiated from a chronically bruised heel (common in fast bowlers and race walkers who tend to stamp the heel down hard) by the hop test, when pain should be worse hopping on the forefoot, while the bruised heel feels easier. There is localized tenderness under the calcaneum. The bruise responds to an injection more posterior in the middle of the heel pad.

Treatment must be directed towards the local pathology, which is an insertional tendinitis at the site of the plantar fascia/bone contact. Subperiosteal infiltration with corticosteroid and lignocaine is the appropriate treatment and, in the presence of a flat foot, exercises should be given to build up the intrinsic musculature of the feet, hopefully preventing a relapse.

### 6.37  What is pes planus and how is it managed?

A common cause of foot pain probably relates to a pes planus or flat foot. The foot has numerous muscles and ligaments and these maintain the normal arch and therefore normal posture and mobility. However, for a variety of reasons ranging from bad footwear to bad luck the arch can be lost and this inevitably strains the ligaments and muscles, which then causes foot pain and stiffness.

Treatment must be directed towards appropriate strengthening exercises, focusing on the intrinsic musculature of the foot. Specifically, I have the patient carry out slow rotational exercises in each direction with attempts at dorsiflexion and plantarflexion, coiling the toes as if to make a 'fist' of the foot and hyperextending the toes, together with inversion and eversion exercises, walking on tiptoes, etc. Local painful ligaments may also benefit from local injection at the site of insertion if there is local pathology.

### 6.38  What are the common problems of the forefoot?

A glomus tumour is situated between the second and third metatarsal bones and can present with pain at rest and on weight-bearing. This is an unusual pathology and usually requires surgical intervention. By contrast, most localized foot problems relate to ligamentous insertion tendinitis or arthropathy at various sites. Given that there are so many small joints in the foot, it is not surprising that a localized monoarthropathy can give trouble and yet be difficult to define in terms of precise location. In order of common problems the first MTP is the most usual site for discomfort. This may present as the classical 'bunion' or may simply be associated with pain and little swelling. Any of the MTP joints can present with localized arthropathy — the patient complaining of a feeling of 'walking on a pebble or pebbles'.

The first MTP joint (the site of the bunion) is frequently a site of degenerative change and may interfere with footwear and often benefit from intra-articular steroid injection. Painful MTPs at other sites can also give trouble, although less frequently.

A hallux rigidus, where extension of the big toe is restricted, may be improved by an injection of steroid into the MTP joint. However, if the degenerative changes are advanced, benefit may be temporary.

### 6.39  What about problems elsewhere in the foot?

Less frequently, problems may be seen in the mid-foot and these may relate to capsular damage or low-grade synovitis of one of the intratarsal joints.

More proximally, the next most common pathology relates to the lateral or medial ankle ligaments where they insert into the hindfoot. In all these ligamentous insertional problems the pathology is analogous to that seen at the lateral or medial epicondyle (tennis or golfer's elbow).

Finally, there may be tenosynovitis of the tendon sheaths of the long extensors of the toes — usually presenting with mid-foot pain on exertion.

### 6.40  What areas of the foot can be injected and what areas should be avoided?

Clearly, all the tenosynovial sheaths can be treated with local injection as can any of the intra-articular problems. Plantar fasciitis, in my experience, only responds to injection. The question could well be phrased: 'What areas should be avoided in terms of injection?'. In fact, it is often the case that when everything else has been tried, it is still worth injecting but obviously this should be performed by a rheumatologist with experience. For example, tarsonavicular or subtalar injections may help greatly but are fairly difficult to perform without a certain amount of experience. In summary, nothing should be avoided.

# 7. Systemic diseases (RA, AS and seronegative arthritides)

This chapter covers rheumatoid arthritis (RA), ankylosing spondylitis (AS) and the other seronegative spondylarthropathies with a focus on psoriatic arthropathy and Reiter's disease. The rare disorders (e.g. systemic lupus erythematosus, progressive systemic sclerosis, etc.) are of relatively little interest to the GP given the few patients that will be seen in any one year with these conditions. We will therefore deal predominantly with rheumatoid disease and the spondylarthropathies. Other generalized joint diseases are covered in Chapter 9.

## RHEUMATOID ARTHRITIS (RA)

### 7.1 What are the important features of RA?

RA is an inflammatory arthropathy and multisystem disease affecting multiple joints usually in a symmetrical manner. Both small and large joints may be involved, and upper and lower limbs are affected equally. Since the condition is a multisystem disorder (see Fig. 2.1), rheumatologists tend to use the term 'rheumatoid disease' rather than rheumatoid arthritis. Virtually every tissue in the body can be involved. The characteristic symptoms are those of pain and swelling of the joints, with stiffness and fatigue.

Over 90% of patients are seropositive for rheumatoid factor, an autoimmune phenomenon.

### 7.2 What is the aetiology of RA?

The disorder is of unknown aetiology although it is clear that genetic factors are relevant and, almost certain, that an infective trigger sets off the disease. This is likely to be a virus and, more specifically, a retrovirus. However, some data support the contention that RA is an 'allergic' response to *Mycobacterium tuberculosis* or a host of other micro-organisms.

## 7.3  Who is affected by this disease?

RA can present at any age. However, there is no doubt that women of childbearing age are most frequently affected. Overall, the sex ratio favours women 3:1 with a ratio that is somewhat less in favour of women in the seventh and eighth decades. Teenage girls can get RA, but the peak is probably in the late thirties and early forties.

Patients may present a clearly defined picture of seropositive rheumatoid disease developing perhaps at the age of 40 years. However, on further discussion it becomes apparent that the individual had a self-limiting inflammatory arthropathy that lasted a few months, some 15 years earlier. In such a situation it is difficult to be sure whether the RA presented early on in the third decade or whether that was a coincidental self-limiting post-viral phenomenon.

A young adult woman or middle-aged woman presenting with a polysynovitis in the absence of obvious viral contact makes one think of RA. If there is quite marked swelling, the diagnosis is even more likely and, of course, if a nodule is seen then RA is almost certainly the diagnosis. In the early stages, radiographs are unhelpful because one would not expect to see erosions until several weeks, if not months, have passed.

**Table 7.1**  Main features of rheumatoid nodules

| Location | Anywhere (found in 30% of seropositive patients) |
|---|---|
| Typical site | Extensor surface of elbows and forearm |
| | Pressure points of feet, buttocks and hands |
| | Usually subcutaneous but may be subperiosteal |
| Complications | Infection |
| | Pain (pressure point) |
| | Ulceration |
| | Rupture of underlying tendons |
| | Functional (depending on location) |
| |     Cardiac conduction defect |
| |     Laryngeal disturbance |
| |     Spinal cord compression |

## 7.4 What are the first symptoms of RA?

RA may present explosively over a few days or insidiously over weeks or months. The most common presentation is that of a polysynovitis affecting small and large joints alike but, occasionally, a patient may present with just one painful wrist and a painful knee, for example, or even an asymmetrical presentation affecting just one side of the body is sometimes seen. Often, associated with the pain and swelling of the joints, there is stiffness and generalized fatigue.

## 7.5 What are the first signs of RA?

The disease is predominantly a synovitis and so soft-tissue swelling directly around the joints can be expected rather than the extra-articular swelling seen in the spondylarthropathies discussed elsewhere.

Extra-articular manifestations can affect almost all the organs of the body. These are summarized in Figure 2.1.

The most common systemic manifestation is fatigue and this, in turn, can relate to the disease itself, in terms of the inflammatory disorder, or to a secondary anaemia. The latter, in turn, can be the anaemia of chronic disease or may be related to an NSAID-induced gastric blood loss.

Rheumatoid nodules frequently occur and again these can be found anywhere. However, the most common location is over pressure sites such as the elbow, Achilles tendon, over the small joints of the hands and other locations (Table 7.1). Other nodules seen in general practice are summarized in Table 7.2.

**Table 7.2** The differential diagnosis of rheumatoid nodules

| Location | Type of nodule |
| --- | --- |
| Lung | Cancer |
| Pinna of ear | Gouty tophi |
| Bridge of nose | Basal cell carcinoma |
| Tendons | Xanthomata |
| Subcutaneous | Tophi |
| | Rheumatic fever nodules |
| | Calcinosis |
| | Xanthomata |
| | Neurofibromata |
| | Epidermal cysts |

**Table 7.3** Comparison of the main features of RA and degenerative joint disease (osteoarthritis)

| Features | Rheumatoid arthritis | Osteoarthritis |
|---|---|---|
| Ethnic distribution | All races | All races |
| Sex ratio (female:male) | 3:1 | Slight female preponderance |
| Age of onset | All ages | Rare before fifth decade |
| Peak incidence (years) | 20–40 | >65 |
| Prevalence | 0.5–1% | Radiological 50% (>60 years) Clinical >10% (>60 years) |
| Systemic disease (constitutional upset) | Yes | No |
| Multisystem disorder | Yes | No |
| Joints affected | All | Weight-bearing, spine, distal interphalangeal, first carpometacarpal joints |
| Symmetry | Symmetrical (80%) | Asymmetrical (90%) |
| Morning stiffness | Marked | Minimal |
| Inflammatory synovitis | 100% | <5% |
| Heberden's nodes (distal interphalangeal) | No | Yes |
| Bouchard's nodes (proximal interphalangeal) | No | Yes |
| Rheumatoid nodules | Yes | No |
| Radiology | Osteoporosis, erosions, joint space loss | Osteosclerosis, new bone formation, joint space loss |
| Rheumatoid factor | Positive ($\approx$ 90%), high titre (usually 1:160) | Positive (<10%), low titre |

## 7.6  What is the differential diagnosis between RA and OA?

The main features of history and presentation are listed in Table 7.3.

## 7.7  What is the role of laboratory investigations in diagnosis?

Regardless of aetiology the disorder is usually easy to recognize and diagnose since most patients are seropositive for rheumatoid factor (IgM anti-IgG antibody). In association with the rheumatoid factor, other laboratory abnormalities occur including a raised erythrocyte sedimentation rate (ESR) or plasma viscosity and often an anaemia with high platelet count.

## 7.8 How useful a test is rheumatoid factor?

The rheumatoid factor is useful in one setting only. In patients with an inflammatory joint disease it is helpful to know whether they are rheumatoid-factor-positive or -negative. In other words, is it a seronegative inflammatory arthritis or classical seropositive RA? Too often we see the test performed for anybody who presents with pain anywhere. It is clearly an expense and it should be realized that some 5% of people are rheumatoid factor-positive unrelated to any joint disease, so we see much undue concern regarding the seropositivity of individuals.

Nevertheless, high titre positivity virtually only occurs in RA itself. Thus, a patient presenting with polysynovitis and a high titre of rheumatoid factor almost certainly has RA and, if the typical erosions are present on the radiograph, the diagnosis is 99.9% certain.

## 7.9 What is the role of radiological investigation?

The only value of the radiograph is if it is going to alter the management of the patient. Is there something that we would see on the radiograph that would make us change our mind in terms of diagnosis or treatment? If it is purely to satisfy the patient or for academic interest then we should avoid the test, which is inevitably time-consuming and expensive. Of course, there are exceptions. For example, when planning surgery or assessing a patient with severe neck pain, a radiograph will be needed. In general, serial films are of limited benefit but may have a minor role to play in the occasional patient with RA when there is uncertainty about disease progression.

## 7.10 How should an early case of widespread RA be managed?

Once the diagnosis has been confirmed with appropriate laboratory tests (e.g. full blood picture, plasma viscosity or ESR and rheumatoid factor) together with radiographs if the disease is already established, the patient must be given information about the disease and misinformation must be corrected. The main thrust of early management must be education to ensure that the patient fully understands what may happen, what is happening and how best the symptoms and signs can be managed by the GP, rheumatologist and other health professionals.

A multidisciplinary approach will be needed with physiotherapist, hydrotherapist, occupational therapist, psychological back-up, orthopaedic input as necessary, and perhaps with help from other members of the team.

Almost all patients will require an NSAID and, as a rheumatologist, I would certainly favour the use of a disease-modifying antirheumatic drug such as methotrexate, sooner rather than later. Indeed, once a definitive diagnosis of seropositive rheumatoid disease is made, I would almost always give both an NSAID and a disease-modifying drug. Exceptions would include those who have only mild disease or are pregnant or intending pregnancy in the near future.

### 7.11  Does whether or not the patient is seropositive affect management?

Very, very little. If patients are seropositive with some generalized joint pain and swelling — that means they have RA — one would be slightly more aggressive starting a disease-modifying agent sooner rather than later. The same individual, if seronegative, may have a self-limiting post-viral arthropathy syndrome and one might be prepared to wait another 6–12 weeks before starting methotrexate, gold or penicillamine.

### 7.12  How does the severity of the disease influence management?

Rheumatoid disease is not a benign, self-limiting arthropathy and once a diagnosis is made my approach is to be aggressive. In a way, the more aggressive we are early on, the less aggressive we will have to be in the future. Clearly, some individuals fail to respond to all conventional drugs and, in such individuals, further aggression in terms of experimental agents will be indicated.

If a patient has seropositive active disease that does not respond adequately to 4–6 weeks of an NSAID, methotrexate or some other disease-modifying drug is introduced. As stressed several times, the sooner powerful medication is introduced the better. Such a patient should be referred urgently to the rheumatologist in order to optimize physiotherapy and hydrotherapy and the other aspects of the multidisciplinary team approach. Current practice is to admit patients as a day case or for a few days in order to provide pulse methylprednisolone therapy and baseline remedial therapy while introducing a new disease-modifying drug.

### 7.13 What is the best advice for patients who have just been diagnosed?

Perhaps the place to start is to advise the patient that everything they have been told by their friends and neighbours should be forgotten and that they need to learn the true facts. Too often the patient has been frightened by 'advice' from sympathetic friends. It is important to begin again and allow the patient to hear the story from a specialist rather than from elsewhere. Patients must be also warned to avoid 'quack' (and often expensive) therapies. They must quickly learn about proven remedies and learn to evaluate other forms of therapy, which are often more expensive and, perhaps, of little value. The 'rules-of-thumb' would be:

1. Do not expect a quick cure.
2. Any drug that is efficacious has the potential for causing toxicity and must be used intelligently and with care.
3. Innumerable diets have been recommended for arthritis. Clearly, if the perfect diet existed, there would only be one that would be recommended! In summary, no diet is better than any other and the patient should have a sensible diet that he or she enjoys. Indeed, I point out to the patient that RA has more or less comparable severity around the world — regardless of diet. Fish-eating Eskimos have severe disease as do vegetarian groups in India or elsewhere!
4. Although often incurable, relentless progression of disease is the exception and not the rule.
5. The majority of patients live a normal life in terms of occupation and family and social activities.

We can give real hope to patients by helping them learn about the disease and how to live within the constraints of the disorder. New treatments are being developed and safer, more efficacious medications are slowly becoming available.

## 7.14 How should the GP work together with the rheumatologist?

There will always be a place for shared care. Specifically, the GP will monitor the day-to-day (or week-to-week) management decisions and the rheumatologist will make him or herself available to give help when either the GP or patient so wishes. Clearly, decisions regarding a disease-modifying drug (i.e. when to start it or stop it) and other important considerations such as whether inpatient management would be appropriate, would require the specialist's input. Additionally, decisions regarding referral to an orthopaedic surgeon or the management of emergency problems would require assessment by the rheumatologist.

The GP should feel free to telephone the consultant at any time. At the Royal National Hospital for Rheumatic Diseases in Bath we may follow a patient on a 6-monthly, yearly or prn basis, depending on the specific requirements of patient and general practitioner. However, we have weekly emergency clinics and injection clinics and so the patient knows that he or she is only 3–4 days away from a hospital consultation. Moreover, we have a 24-hour telephone help-line.

Ideally, the patient should be seen by the rheumatologist once or twice per year in order to keep at least a distant eye on the changing nature of the disease. However, that may not be possible either because of the distance between the patient and the unit or because the disorder is mild. In such cases the GP can decide when a further referral is required.

## 7.15 How should an established case of RA be managed?

If the patient is losing ground or is developing side-effects on the established therapy, decisions must be taken as to whether the patient would benefit from admission for a thorough review of the whole picture. Alternatively, an outpatient decision can be made about simply changing the disease-modifying drug from one to another. The skill in managing established rheumatoid disease is to anticipate problems before they arise. For example, it is always better for the hand surgeon to assess the patient with poor hand function and possible tendon damage before an emergency arises resulting in a finger drop or wrist drop.

## 7.16 How best would the GP share care at this stage?

If the disease is stable then the GP can continue to follow the patient without input from the rheumatologist. As mentioned elsewhere, in an ideal situation I would see the patient once every 12 months or so but this is not necessary if there are no therapy changes and if the patient feels that everything is stable.

## 7.17 How should a late or advanced case of RA be managed?

Decisions will need to be made as to whether surgical intervention is appropriate. It may be a matter of admitting the patient for a few days to optimize physio- and hydrotherapy and to see how well the patient can cope without a new knee or hip. By contrast, the multidisciplinary team may reach the conclusion that surgical intervention is required and onward referral would then be necessary.

## 7.18 What is the role of the GP in this situation?

The main role of the GP in advanced rheumatoid disease is to advise the rheumatologist as soon as possible if the patient appears to be deteriorating. Although it is better to be proactive than only to respond to the crises, this is 'easier said than done' in everyday clinical practice. Therefore, sometimes patients are seen who should have been referred a few months earlier. If one waits until the individual has taken to bed and become more-or-less chair- or bed-bound, it is too late.

## 7.19 How does HIV infection complicate the picture?

There is an intricate relationship between HIV and AIDS on the one hand and rheumatology on the other. For example, in the UK one of the commonest forms of presentation of AIDS — at least to the rheumatologist — is by way of a septic arthritis. By contrast, in the USA, AIDS patients may first present to the casualty department with an acute-onset polyarthralgia — polyarthritis syndrome — which can be excruciatingly painful and, interestingly, short lived. Within 4–5 weeks on adequate NSAID therapy, the acute problem melts away. In addition, and again more frequently in the USA than in the UK, patients with HIV can present with a reactive arthritis related to *Chlamydia* spp. or one of the bowel organisms.

Of even greater interest is the fact that patients with RA who coincidentally develop HIV infection tend to enter remission in terms of the rheumatological disease. The reason for this is that the HIV infection destroys the CD4-positive lymphocyte cells — the very cells that are central in maintaining disease activity in rheumatoid disease.

### 7.20  Should a patient get a disease-modifying agent from his or her GP?

There is no reason why not, if the GP is experienced and interested in rheumatology. Often it is a good basis on which to have shared care. The consultant rheumatologist can see the patient once, agree with the GP on the right disease-modifying agent and then perhaps not see the patient again or only perhaps every year or two.

### 7.21  What is the place of the orthopaedic surgeon and other specialities in the management of rheumatoid disease?

Orthopaedic surgeons will be required to replace hips, knees and, with increasing frequency, ankles, shoulders, elbows and other joints. Neurosurgeons may be required to provide help in cervical spine involvement with cord or nerve root entrapment. The hand surgeon or microvascular surgeon (or plastic surgeon) may be needed for tendon grafting in the hands and other complicated localized surgical intervention. The neurologist may have input to determine whether the neurological disability relates to the rheumatoid neck or whether there is a separate explanation for the neurodeficit.

### 7.22  What is it about admission to hospital that makes patients get better so quickly?

There are many ways of answering this question. First, patients frequently benefit by the very fact that the medical profession appears to be taking them seriously. That in itself is of benefit to the patient and has the inevitable additional benefit that home stresses are relieved and that all of us can take extra time to study the clinical situation. Rest itself has a definite 'anti-inflammatory' effect and rheumatologists, for example, have seen the very sick RA patient with widespread systemic involvement coming into hospital for assessment (e.g. regarding more powerful medication) where within 48 hours the entire clinical situation has modified and the active inflamed joints have settled without any drug intervention. It is also evident that when some patients see other individuals who are even sicker and in greater pain, this can have a beneficial effect on their approach to their own problem.

## ANKYLOSING SPONDYLITIS (AS)

### 7.23  What do the terms 'spondylosis' and 'spondylitis' signify?

These two terms are confusing and should be avoided. In theory, spondylosis refers to degenerative changes of the vertebrae, while spondylitis suggests inflammatory disease. However, there is no standardization and their use is unhelpful. For example, when patients learn that their neck radiograph reveals 'spondylitis' or 'spondylosis', they may fear the worst and may confuse the term with AS.

### 7.24  What are the important features of AS?

AS is an inflammatory spinal disease with involvement of the sacroiliac joints and, to a varying degree, ascending spinal disease, extraspinal articular disease and extra-articular systemic symptoms and signs (e.g. iritis, anaemia, aortitis, etc.). AS is the major spondylarthropathy. It is associated with decreased mobility of the lumbar spine in all directions and usually the absence of localized trigger sites on examination. Back pain is the main symptom and must be differentiated from non-specific mechanical back pain problems mentioned in Chapter 4. A comparison of the main features of AS and RA is shown in Table 7.4.

### 7.25  What is the aetiology of AS?

AS itself is known as primary (i.e. in the absence of any other aetiological factor) or secondary to psoriasis, inflammatory bowel

**Table 7.4** Comparison between AS and RA in both men and women

| Features | Rheumatoid arthritis | Ankylosing spondylitis | |
|---|---|---|---|
| | | Men | Women |
| Prevalence | 0.5–1% | 0.5% | 0.2% |
| Age of onset (years) | All ages | 20–40 | 20–40 |
| Peak incidence (years) | 20–40 | 20–30 | 20–30 |
| Family clustering | Rare | Common | Common |
| HLA-B27 | 6% (normal) | 95% | 95% |
| HLA-DR4 | 60% | 25% (normal) | 25% (normal) |
| Rheumatoid factor | ≈ 90% | 5% | 5% |
| Rheumatoid nodules | Yes | No | No |
| Peripheral joint disease | 100% | 20% | 40% |
| Spinal symptoms | Cervical only (rare) | Present (often severe) | Present (often mild) |
| Radiology | | | |
| Sacroiliitis | 0% | 100% | 100% |
| Spinal disease (syndesmophytes) | 0% | 50% | 25% |
| Classical bamboo spine | No | Common | Rare |

disease or reactive arthropathy/Reiter's disease). Well over 95% of Caucasian cases with primary disease are HLA B27-positive, while some 80% of those with secondary forms are HLA B27-positive — a genetic marker that is present in some 5–10% of the normal white UK population. Comparable figures for the black population in the UK are around 50% and 4%, respectively.

## 7.26  Who is affected by this disease?

AS affects up to 0.5% of the population. It typically occurs during the second and third decades. The development of AS after the age of 30 or 35 years is extremely unusual.

## 7.27 What are the main presenting features?

There are five major factors:

1. Age at onset is invariably below the age of 40 years.
2. Onset of the pain is insidious, developing over weeks or even months rather than on a specific day.
3. Pain has usually been present for at least 3 months before the physician is first contacted. This relates to the fact that the onset is mild and barely noticeable for the first weeks.

4. Pain is worst in the morning, associated with morning stiffness and improves during the day.
5. Perhaps most important of all, the pain is worsened by rest and improves with exercise.

If three or more of these features are present then a plain antero-posterior radiograph of the pelvis should be done. This will define whether sacroiliitis is present (i.e. AS) or otherwise. Within days of beginning an NSAID there should be a major improvement in pain and movement.

Tables 7.5 and 7.6 summarize the diagnostic and clinical criteria for AS.

**Table 7.5** Criteria for diagnosing AS (Rome, 1961)

| Clinical criteria | Radiological criterion |
|---|---|
| Low back pain and stiffness for more than 3 months that is not relieved by rest | Radiograph showing bilateral sacroiliac changes characteristic of ankylosing spondylitis (this would exclude bilateral osteoarthrosis of the sacroiliac joints) |
| Pain and stiffness in the thoracic region | |
| Limited motion in the lumbar spine | |
| Limited chest expansion | |
| History or evidence of iritis or its sequelae | |

**Table 7.6** Clinical criteria for AS (New York, 1966)

| Diagnosis | Grading |
|---|---|
| Limitation of motion of the lumbar spine in all three planes — anterior flexion, lateral flexion and extension | *Definite*<br>Grade 3–4 bilateral sacroiliitis with at least one clinical criterion |
| History or the presence of pain at the dorsolumbar junction or in the lumbar spine | Grade 3–4 unilateral or grade 2 bilateral sacroiliitis with clinical criterion 1 (limitation of back movement in all three planes) or with both clinical criteria 2 and 3 (back pain and limitation of chest expansion) |
| Limitation of chest expansion to 1 inch (2. 5 cm) or less, measured at the level of the fourth intercostal space | *Probable*<br>Grade 3–4 bilateral sacroiliitis with no clinical criteria |

## 7.28 It often takes a long time for a GP to make the diagnosis of AS, sometimes many years; how can this be improved?

Worldwide studies have shown a delay in men of up to 7 or 8 years and in women of up to 10 years before the diagnosis is made. There are several reasons for this. First, AS was considered to be rare in women and therefore it was natural to assume that back pain in a women related to non-specific problems rather than AS. In fact, we now recognize that some 30–40% of patients with AS are women and so our index of suspicion must be high in both sexes. The second reason is that back pain is extraordinarily common in general and AS relatively rare. It is easy to forget about AS. The third point is that the early symptoms are very mild and therefore patients often learn to live with their symptoms rather than persist in trying to reach a diagnosis. Furthermore, many patients will visit an osteopath, chiropractitioner or other complementary practitioners rather than the GP. Lastly, even when the patient with persistent pain does see the GP and even if a radiograph of the sacroiliac joints are requested, radiologists sometimes miss the diagnosis unless the sacroiliac joints are totally fused.

Fortunately, now with the increased interest in AS and pressure from the patient group known as the National Ankylosing Spondylitis Society (see Appendix 1 for details), all practitioners and radiologists are becoming more aware of the problem and it is hoped that the diagnosis will be reached sooner rather than later.

## 7.29 Why do some patients with AS get a sudden flare-up of their back pain?

At any stage in the course of primary AS or secondary forms (related to psoriasis, inflammatory bowel disease, etc.) patients may develop an acute exacerbation of back pain, often related to ligamentous insertion inflammation. This site, where ligaments infiltrate into bone, is known as the enthesis and, for reasons that are unclear, inflammation at this site is the characteristic pathology in the spondylarthritides. This explains why some patients present with chest pain of a more-or-less pleuritic nature. It would appear that the intercostal muscles develop enthesopathic change at the site of insertion of the ligament into bone and thus deep inspiration results in chest wall pain. In addition, costochondritis occurs in AS as a cause of localized chest wall pain.

### 7.30  When should infective sacroiliitis be considered?

There can be the very rare case of a septic sacroiliitis, rather than the non-infective inflammatory sacroiliitis of AS. The infective variety presents typically in young children below the age of 10 years. Symptoms may be dramatic and sudden with high fever and extreme pain on movement. In such small children 'stressing' the pelvis may cause an acute exacerbation of pain. A radiograph may reveal diffuse loss of density around the joint in an asymmetrical fashion. Blood cultures and a needle aspiration of the sacroiliac joint is of paramount importance to define the precise organism with sensitivities. This allows the appropriate use of an antibiotic.

### 7.31  What is the management of AS?

AS is a relatively simple condition to manage given the response to NSAIDs and a correct exercise programme.

The patient should be educated as to the nature of the condition and given appropriate advice regarding the exercise programme that should be followed indefinitely.

In general, patients are encouraged to stop smoking and to begin exercise. Swimming is best. Close attention to posture is important. One pillow at night is the maximum support needed. A firm mattress is appropriate. In addition, an NSAID (e.g. indomethacin 75 mg slow-release once each night or twice daily) will decrease pain and stiffness.

In addition a booklet is available, which contains the name and address of the National AS Society, which the patients are encouraged to join. This will provide them with further information regarding their condition. Patients can be given leaflets on the National Osteoporosis Society and this again includes some basic information on posture and back pain. The Back Pain Association can also provide literature for patients and all the appropriate addresses and contact numbers are given in the appendix. In terms of those patients referred to hospital, physiotherapists can provide additional leaflets regarding patients' specific problems and the appropriate exercise programme. This is certainly an area that needs to be explored so that more appropriate material can become available for practitioners to distribute to their patients. As an example, for those patients who do have AS we have prepared a booklet that addresses the background and management programme (available from the National Ankylosing Spondylitis Society — see Appendix 1).

## SERONEGATIVE ARTHRITIDES

### 7.32  What seronegative arthritic conditions may exist?

Apart from AS, the other seronegative spondylarthritides are psoriatic spondylitis, Reiter's syndrome (and the other reactive arthritides) and enteropathic arthropathy (following Crohn's disease and ulcerative colitis). In addition, there are many other forms of seronegative arthritis including seronegative RA, viral arthropathy, chronic pyrophosphate arthropathy and other rarer conditions.

### 7.33  How would you set about elucidating these?

The seronegative arthridites tend to present with peripheral joint disease rather than spinal involvement *per se*. However, there are exceptions, and we certainly see patients with psoriasis, Reiter's and the other entities presenting initially with back pain. Interestingly, the juvenile-onset spondylarthropathy syndrome tends again to present with peripheral joint disease and even juvenile AS, itself, rarely presents with back pain.

Therefore, in patients with peripheral joint or spinal disease the other entities should be considered and a family history taken for psoriasis and inflammatory bowel disease. The patient must be questioned and examined closely regarding psoriasis or other problems. For example, when examining the patient, a close search would be made for scalp psoriasis, psoriatic nail disease and other evidence of psoriasis in hidden areas such as the gluteal cleft or umbilicus. In addition, patients will be questioned as to the presence or otherwise of diarrhoea or mucus in the stool. Even a mild change in bowel habit may be sufficient to bring some enteropathic arthritis to the attention of the physician. Urethritis, cervicitis, vaginal discharge, urinary frequency and urgency are all symptoms present in sexually acquired (and occasional postintestinal) Reiter's disease.

In general, no additional investigations are required in patients with secondary forms of spondylitis, unless symptoms or signs direct attention towards a specific area. For example, if an individual has diarrhoea or mucus in the stool then investigation for inflammatory bowel disease would be appropriate. This could include sigmoidoscopy and ileocolonoscopy.

## 7.34 What is the management of the seronegative spondylarthritides?

In general, treatment is directed both at the AS itself and at the primary condition. For example, if the patient has enteropathic spondylitis then the bowel inflammation must be controlled with sulphasalazine or other agents. There are two rheumatological manifestations of inflammatory bowel disease. The first is that of an acute peripheral synovitis (typically the knee or ankle) in association with active severe inflammatory bowel disease. In such a situation the joint problem usually settles as the bowel disease is treated. In contrast, the spinal disease complicating inflammatory bowel disease continues unabated regardless of whether the bowel disease is (or is not) suppressed. Naturally, treatment should be directed at both systems separately for the benefit of the patient.

With psoriatic spondylarthropathy, again the psoriasis should be treated separately from the spinal condition. However, with peripheral joint involvement, methotrexate may be the drug of choice both for the psoriasis and for the peripheral joints. To what extent such an agent improves the spinal symptoms is unclear.

With reactive arthropathy/Reiter's disease complicated by AS, treatment is directed towards the spine together with local injections for the peripheral joints, NSAIDs and appropriate spinal exercises. When necessary, methotrexate is added.

# 8. Osteoarthritis

Osteoarthritis (OA), also known as osteoarthropathy or degenerative joint disease, is a mixed bag of end-stage arthropathies loosely lumped together by the title 'osteoarthritis'. The condition should be considered as 'joint failure' analogous to heart failure. The different aspects of this condition will be discussed and the particular features of this disease in certain locations (e.g. hip only, distal interphalangeal joints only, etc.) will be highlighted.

## 8.1 What is the current definition of OA?

There is no clear definition of OA. OA is used interchangeably with the term osteoarthrosis and degenerative joint disease and joint failure. The first refers to the concept that there is an inflammatory component in degenerative joint disease, while osteoarthrosis is the label favoured by those who feel that the process is purely mechanical and 'degenerative'. Degenerative joint disease is widely used and avoids the debate as to whether the ending should be -osis or -itis. However, some of us prefer the concept of 'regenerative' joint disease rather than 'degenerative' given the new bone formation, the juxta-articular sclerosis and the recognized pathological evidence of repair. It may be that symptoms only become evident when the regenerative change cannot suffice in terms of the ongoing damage.

Osteoarthropathy (my preferred term given that this avoids any of the above disagreement and is perhaps the most 'open-minded' of the labels) can be defined in a variety of ways. None is perfect and there are clearly inconsistencies with any of the definitions.

## 8.2 What is the aetiology of OA?

Perhaps the best way of thinking of OA is analogous to the label 'heart failure', which is the end point of a variety of aetiologies, such as ischaemic heart disease, valvular heart disease, hypertensive heart disease, etc. Similarly, a variety of entities can result in so called OA. The most common aetiology relates to cartilage failure of unknown cause. However, there are clearly genetic factors, and acquired factors such as trauma, inflammatory disease, misalignment, etc.

### 8.3  Who is affected?

OA can present at any age in a patient with a genetically determined collagen anomaly, developmental change or following a traumatic or other destructive episode to the joint. However, typically patients are in their sixth or seventh decade when they first become aware of the more common form of degenerative disease. There are exceptions such as the Heberden's and Bouchard's nodes that are often familial in nature and may arise during the fourth or fifth decade or even earlier. Daughters and nieces of patients with disease are at risk of developing a similar problem at a comparable age.

There is a suggestion that 80- and 90-year-olds are rather less likely to develop disease than are those 10 or 20 years younger. This phenomenon may be spurious in that it could be that individuals who survive that long without disease are less at risk of developing arthropathy — but it might be that degenerative arthropathy itself is associated in some way with shorter survival. In other words, it is just possible that OA predicts earlier death — and, conversely, absence of OA is associated with longevity.

### 8.4  Are sports professionals, such as footballers, particularly at risk?

This question has intrigued epidemiologists and rheumatologists for decades. Perhaps some of the best studies have related to long-distance runners. In such individuals it is apparent that the amount of radiological change is greater in those who continue to run, in contrast to an age-matched control group who is sedentary in nature. However, symptoms emanating from the knee are greater in the controls who have little exercise than in those who have run, on average, 50 km per week. This immediately tells us that there is a dissociation between radiological change and symptoms — a phenomenon that we already recognize and have discussed elsewhere. Thus, to answer the question, it has to be accepted that repetitive exercising can cause changes that are recognized radiologically but it would appear that symptoms are *not* more prevalent. To extrapolate from such well-controlled studies to other sporting activities such as football is not easy. We do know whether major trauma with capsular damage and perhaps fractures that enter the joint relate to later OA but the repeated microtrauma of the average footballer does not appear to have a major affect on ankle or knee joints. Indeed, studies of professional footballers have revealed little in the way of radiological or symptomatic change unless major traumatic episodes have occurred.

By contrast, if we consider those who spend their life parachute jumping, ankle osteoarthropathy secondary to repeated major traumata at the ankle is a real phenomenon.

Individuals who use other joints in a repetitive nature are at greater risk of some degenerative change and we have certainly commented in the past on so-called game-keeper's thumb! This is an osteoarthropathy affecting the first carpometacarpal joint in an individual who continuously strains his thumb breaking the neck of wild animals!

## 8.5  Is there anything that can be done to avoid OA?

No. Nevertheless, having said that, keeping the musculature strong in proximity to those joints that are at risk is certainly good in terms of long-term symptoms. As discussed above, the long-distance runner has fewer symptoms than a sedentary individual. Swimming is also an excellent sport in as much as this builds up the musculature, which, in turn, protects the joints. Regular quadriceps exercises is an excellent way to decrease knee symptoms and so although OA — in radiological terms — cannot be prevented, many of the symptoms can.

Another important point is that as society becomes generally more healthy and fitter, there will be more complaints related to the locomotor system. Obviously, a chair-bound individual with end-stage heart failure is going to be unaware of a painful knee or hip. It is only the relatively fit who expect to continue to be active who are more likely to complain.

## 8.6 What are the first symptoms?

Stiffness following rest is perhaps the first problem that the patient will notice. There may be effusions — particularly in the knee or localized tenderness at the site of ligamentous insertion into bone. For instance, medial knee pain may relate to the insertion of the medial collateral ligament, while lateral knee pain can be caused by damage to the insertion of the lateral collateral ligament — a phenomenon analogous to medial or lateral epicondylitis at the elbow. In both cases, such pathology can relate to degenerative change, effusions of the knee, weak quadriceps, poor knee support and more strain on either medial or lateral ligaments.

In general the symptoms depend on the site. First carpometacarpal joint arthropathy usually presents early on with pain, whereas hip arthritis may present with stiffness or deteriorating function rather than pain. (See Table 7.3 for a comparison between the main features of RA and OA.)

## 8.7 What are the presenting features that favour a diagnosis of OA?

In general the physician has a high index of suspicion for OA given its extraordinarily high prevalence. In a patient who is over the age of 60 years presenting with pain at the base of the thumb, degenerative joint disease is the correct diagnosis '99 times out of 100'. In a patient with a painful knee, particularly on walking downstairs (e.g. patellofemoral osteoarthropathy) the diagnosis is OA of the patellofemoral compartment unless the individual is below the age of 40–50 years.

OA of the distal and proximal interphalangeal joints (Heberden's nodes and Bouchard's nodes, respectively) may present simply with unsightly deformity rather than symptoms, which can come later. Naturally there are no clinical signs of hip disease until the mobility has decreased and the physician may then note decrease in internal rotation of the hip, decreased extension or at a later stage external rotation. Knee osteoarthritis may be apparent when the physician notes either weak quadriceps apparatus or a small effusion.

## 8.8 How is the diagnosis of OA confirmed?

By definition, osteoarthropathy can be defined either in terms of radiological or pathological change. Clearly we are not going to get a biopsy on every painful joint and so a radiographic examination will be required to be fully certain.

Clinical features are a painful joint, sometimes with swelling and deformity and no diagnostic label such as crystal-induced arthropathy, septic arthropathy, internal derangement, rheumatoid disease, etc. There may be a varying degree of joint deformity. There is universal agreement that the characteristic radiological changes include juxta-articular sclerosis, joint-space narrowing as the cartilage is destroyed, osteophytosis and perhaps erosions. However, osteoarthritis is not necessarily the cause of the symptoms since the pain may emanate from elsewhere and the radiographic change may be irrelevant. Pathologically, OA can be defined in terms of recognized cartilage and bone changes with a low-grade synovial inflammatory reaction.

By contrast, rheumatoid disease would be characterized radiologically by juxta-articular osteoporosis rather than sclerosis, the absence of new bone formation, erosive disease affecting bone and, perhaps, cartilage damage with joint deformity.

## 8.9  How should an early case of OA be managed?

In general terms, the patient must be reassured that OA is not necessarily a chronic deteriorating condition. Most patients can be helped with: (1) simple advice about appropriate exercises (for example quadriceps exercises); (2) the use of simple analgesics; (3) local corticosteroid injections; (4) the use of a cane (walking stick) in the contralateral hand in the case of hip OA ; and/or (5) appropriate use of NSAIDs.

## 8.10  When is referral appropriate?

For patients with widespread intractable disease, review by a rheumatologist would be appropriate and it may even be sensible to admit the patient for a few days for an aggressive rehabilitation programme. In general, the rheumatologist can be called upon for complicated procedures such as an intra-articular steroid injection into the hip, which may decrease the need for future hip arthroplasty.

## 8.11  What hopeful advice can patients be given?

The most important point is that OA is not always a relentlessly progressive disease. We can stress that even if it does progress relentlessly, hip and knee replacements are an excellent therapeutic option. Localized OA rarely spreads to other parts of the body. Although there is a genetic component, bad disease in the father or mother does not imply a similar bad story for the offspring.

With regards to treatment, OA is not fatal but NSAIDs and other medical approaches to therapy may be! In other words, patients must be aware that it is important sometimes to put up with a few symptoms to avoid any sinister side-effect of drugs. Of course NSAIDs have their place but they are not the total answer. Patients must be advised to build up the musculature in such a way that joints can be protected.

### 8.12  How would straightforward OA of the knee be treated?

First, the patient must be reassured that many of the symptoms can be decreased using simple modalities. Clearly, not everyone needs a total knee replacement and equally clearly, the radiological evidence of degenerative arthropathy cannot be cured. Nevertheless, the symptoms can be greatly eased.

Attention must be directed towards the quadriceps apparatus. The more support the knee gets from these muscles, the fewer the symptoms. In general, 80% of knee support comes not from the structure of the knee but from the muscles, in contrast to other joints where the architecture of the joint plays the major role in joint function and support.

Once the muscles are built up, symptoms will often subside. Intra-articular steroid injections into the knee may reduce the synovial reaction and break the vicious cycle. Simple analgesics followed, where necessary, by NSAIDs may be appropriate. In general, only short courses of NSAIDs should be given and the patient warned of the potential side-effects associated with this class of drug.

### 8.13  How would patellofemoral pain be treated?

The mainstay of treatment in such a situation is quadriceps exercises, at first without and then with weights. The quadriceps apparatus must be built up, which in turn lifts the patella away from the knee and reduces the symptoms.

## 8.14  How should a patient with degenerative arthropathy of the knee who is not bad enough for surgery but does not respond adequately to conservative therapy be treated?

We often favour the idea of an arthroscopic lavage in such patients. For reasons that are not well understood, running 1 litre of saline into the knee through the lateral or medial compartment and draining the fluid through the contralateral compartment has a very beneficial effect that may last months or even longer. There are various reasons why this lavage should help. First, as the procedure is carried out, much detritus is seen exuding from the knee. This is a mixture of clots, debris, crystal and other unwanted material. It is also possible that the cold fluid itself has a beneficial effect. Regardless of how lavage works, patients are often delighted with the outcome and frequently request a similar procedure on the contralateral side.

To carry out an arthroscopic lavage, patients are usually admitted as a day case for 3–4 hours. The procedure may take 60 minutes and the patient is then kept in for about 3 hours with a tight dressing, which is released before the patient leaves. The procedure is carried out under local anaesthetic and no sutures are needed — butterflies suffice for the tiny incision.

## 8.15  When should the patient be referred to an orthopaedic surgeon?

The only point in referring the patient to an orthopaedic surgeon is if the GP feels that a new joint is required or that another form of surgical intervention is going to be needed. Most individuals with OA do not require a new hip or a new knee.

## 8.16  How would a late case of widespread OA be managed?

First the patient should be reassured that there is still something we can do to help. This may simply be a matter of remedial exercises to enhance what musculature is still present and to protect the joints. Alternatively, it may be a question of showing the patient how to carry out functions that are not easy because of joint damage, where, with a few tricks, the same procedure can be performed quite simply.

Naturally, patients with widespread disease cannot be expected to respond to local corticosteroid therapy and for such individuals NSAIDs will often be needed. However, particular care must be taken in the older population.

## 8.17  How would the GP liaise with the rheumatologist in the care of such a patient?

It is important for the GP to know exactly what the rheumatologist can and cannot do. It may be that, with the multidisciplinary approach in hospital, a great deal can be done. In addition, the rheumatologist must know from the GP about the home situation and work out realistic goals.

## 8.18  How is treatment tailored to the severity of the disease?

At one end of the spectrum, detailed discussion with the surgeon is appropriate in order to determine whether first the hip should be replaced and then one knee or perhaps both knees (or any other permutation). In such a situation the orthopaedic surgeon, rheumatologist and physiotherapist can get together and discuss the optimum approach. For those with milder disease, joint protection can be taught by the occupational therapists and physiotherapists.

## 8.19  Are there any new treatments for OA just around the corner?

Almost certainly the answer has to be no. Nevertheless, there is a great deal of excitement about agents that could possibly cause cartilage to grow rather than wither, drugs that can decrease the destructive activity of synovial fluid — and even attempts at cartilage replacement are being considered.

It would be unrealistic to think that any magical treatment will become available for at least the next 5–10 years, and then only if we are very lucky.

## 8.20  Are any NSAIDs better than others in OA?

As discussed elsewhere, the better the non-steroidal and the more powerful the analgesic (e.g. indomethacin) the better the symptomatic relief. It may be just this individual who is then going out to play football with little concern and will, in turn, damage the already damaged hip to a greater degree. However, all this is theoretical and there is no generally accepted hard evidence that any one non-steroidal agent is better or worse than another (see Chapter 11).

# 9. Other generalized joint diseases (crystal, metabolic, bone and infective disorders)

This chapter focuses on crystal disorders, Paget's disease, metabolic bone disorders and osteoporosis, together with the infective arthritides.

## GOUT AND OTHER CRYSTAL DISEASES

### 9.1 What are the important features of gout?

Gout is an acute, outstandingly painful, self-limiting but dramatic monosynovitis usually affecting the ankle, knee or first metatarsophalangeal joint. Very occasionally, two or more joints are involved. The attack usually comes on over 2–3 hours, reaching a crescendo within 12 hours, and remitting without therapy over the next 7–10 days. Usually the disease is very sensitive to high-dose NSAIDs — low doses having little effect.

### 9.2 What is the aetiology?

Hyperuricaemia is caused by excess production (genetic defect) or by poor renal excretion (renal dysfunction *or* diuretic therapy). If hyperuricaemia persists and renal function becomes compromised (e.g. lactic acid load following alcohol ingestion), urate crystals can come out of solution and precipitate in synovial fluid causing an acute joint.

### 9.3 How is gout identified?

One of the confusions in practice is that it is very common to see patients who are hyperuricaemic, particularly those who are overweight, hyperlipidaemic, a bit hypertensive and perhaps who drink heavily. Although they may have joint pains, it is wrong to assume that the hyperuricaemia is causing the symptoms. The majority of patients on a diuretic will be hyperuricaemic but again few of these have gout. The advantage of putting a needle into a joint and finding crystals is that a definitive diagnosis can be made. Otherwise the evidence is only circumstantial. In an acute attack, the reddened joint will be extremely tender and, over the ensuing hours, the skin may flake — an important finding in acute gout. Only a septic joint can mimic these symptoms and signs.

Apart from the characteristic symptoms and signs, the uric acid level is almost immaterial. In general, hyperuricaemia should be ignored and not treated but it should be simply thought of as a good marker for obesity, hyperlipidaemia, excess alcohol and so on, and these factors should be addressed.

### 9.4  What is the management of gout?

There are two major factors in the management of the patient with gout. First, the diagnosis must be definitive and second, it must be clear whether one is treating the acute attack or attempting to prevent future attacks. Only the presence of urate crystals can substantiate that gout is the diagnosis. Having confirmed a diagnosis of gout, the acute attack is treated with high-dose NSAIDs. My approach would be to give indomethacin 100 mg immediately and repeat this with 50 mg four times in the first day, followed by a total of 200 mg on the second day, 100 mg the third day and a slow taper thereafter over 10–14 days. A common mistake is to give an NSAID correctly but at too low a dose. Clearly a fragile individual would require a somewhat lower dose. Once the acute attack has settled there may not be another for months or years. Assuming that the patient is hyperuricaemic, the cause of this is addressed and the patient is encouraged to lose weight, have a healthier diet and drink less alcohol. Hypertension or other factors would also be addressed. If a second or third attack appears within a few weeks or months, probenecid should be considered to increase the urinary output of urate or allopurinol to dampen down the urate production. Unfortunately, too many patients are receiving allopurinol unnecessarily in spite of its cost and potential toxicity.

In individuals who require long-term allopurinol, it is of paramount importance to wait for the acute attack to settle and then to cover the introduction of allopurinol for at least 6 weeks with a low dose of a non-steroidal agent, such as indomethacin 25 mg twice a day or 25 mg at night. Without NSAID cover, there is a risk of precipitating an acute flare of gouty arthritis. For patients who, at presentation, already have evidence of urate deposits in the skin (e.g. gouty tophi), allopurinol would be introduced immediately after the acute attack settles. Likewise for those with compromised renal function allopurinol may be introduced sooner rather than later. Intra-articular steroid is always of value for acute gout.

By contrast, pyrophosphate deposition disease (see later) may settle with an NSAID or intra-articular corticosteroid. There are no disease-modifying regimens and allopurinol clearly would be of no value in such patients.

### 9.5  When should allopurinol be given for gout?

In general, if a patient has two or more attacks of acute gout in a 12-month period then allopurinol should be given to decrease the rate at which gouty attacks occur. Secondly, if the patient has chronic tophaceous gout, a phenomenon seen relatively rarely now, that patient should also be given allopurinol. Thirdly, if a patient has one or two attacks of gout and poor renal function, and you are concerned about the hyperuricaemia resulting in further renal damage or renal stones, then allopurinol should be given. In general, too many patients are on allopurinol unnecessarily.

### 9.6  What about other forms of crystal disease?

After gout (urate), there is pseudogout (calcium pyrophosphate deposition disease) and calcium hydroxyapatite crystals.

Pseudogout may take several different forms. For example:

1. There may be an acute gout-like disease, typically occurring in the knee in sicker, older patients (often immediately postoperatively).
2. We also recognize a more generalized, less acute, inflammatory arthropathy sometimes known as 'pseudorheumatoid-like

arthropathy', affecting wrists and even smaller joints.

3. Pyrophosphate deposition may cause an accelerated degenerative arthropathic process.

4. It may be a chance radiological finding with deposition in hyaline — and fibrocartilage. This is called chondrocalcinosis.

Calcium hydroxyapatite crystals may occur as a chance radiological appearance or may be associated with a severe acute calcific tendinitis, as discussed in Chapter 5.

## PAGET'S DISEASE AND METABOLIC BONE DISORDERS

### 9.7  What are the important features of Paget's disease?

Paget's disease is a relatively common disorder affecting up to 5% of the UK population. Interestingly, this is relatively high compared with other communities. For example, in the southern USA, Paget's disease is almost unknown.

In Paget's disease there is abnormal turnover of bone and although the bone may be apparently more sclerotic, the quality of the bone is poor and fractures may occur. The disease can be defined in terms of radiological change or pathology. In general, Paget's disease does not hurt unless deformity develops with the inevitable strain on adjoining tissue. Secondly, if Paget's disease enters into the joint then secondary arthropathy can develop. Most cases of Paget's disease are, however, clinically silent and a chance radiological finding. The older textbooks suggested that a requirement for increasing hat size was a good pointer towards the possibility of Paget's disease.

If Paget's disease is suspected, and if it is symptomatic and requiring therapy, it is worthwhile measuring alkaline phosphatase and urinary hydroxyproline — both of which will be raised in active Paget's disease.

### 9.8  How is Paget's disease managed?

The majority of patients require no treatment or merely an NSAID. For those with intractable pain that does not respond to an

NSAID, bisphosphonates or calcitonin are appropriate therapies.

### 9.9  Are osteomalacia and rickets still seen in the UK?

Osteomalacia is becoming more rather than less common. This relates to the ethnic change within the UK. Those with dark skin — especially when living in the north of the country — are particularly at risk from osteomalacia. This must always be considered in the differential diagnosis of patients presenting with bone pain and malaise. The same comments apply to rickets, although this is becoming less frequent as dietary sources of vitamin D are usually adequate in the young.

### 9.10  How is osteomalacia diagnosed and managed?

Osteomalacia is easily missed. The most important factor in the diagnosis of osteomalacia is to remember the features of the at-risk groups (i.e. a non-Caucasian individual with poor diet or a sick older patient with inadequate diet and poverty, etc.). Alkaline phosphatase will be raised and the calcium and phosphate may be low. Radiologically there may be evidence of Looser's fractures and osteoporosis.

Osteomalacia is managed with low-dose vitamin D and attention to renal function.

### 9.11  How do cases of parathyroid bone disease present?

Hyperparathyroidism can present to the GP or rheumatologist with a fibromyalgia-like disease. The same is true of *hypothyroidism* and so the clinician must be prepared to think of these relatively rare (but readily treatable) conditions. Tests for serum calcium and thyroid function would be appropriate for assessing patients who present with widespread poorly defined pain syndromes.

### 9.12  How should hyperparathyroidism and hypothyroidism be managed?

Management is with: (a) parathyroidectomy; and (b) thyroid replacement, respectively.

### 9.13  What are the causes and risk factors of osteoporosis?

Osteoporosis may be defined as too little mineral content in the bone. It is the end result of either too great a loss of mineral or a failure to produce enough in the first place. The final amount of bone stock at its peak is, in turn, an expression of both genetic and environmental factors. Certain races (black) have higher bone mineral content than others (e.g. Asians or whites). This relates to genetic factors but, in addition, we know that in individuals living in an area where there is a high calcium intake, higher bone mineral content is found. Even those individuals who have a high normal bone mineral content may still be at risk for osteoporosis if they are rapid losers, and little is understood about what determines the rate of loss of bone mineral content apart from the factors mentioned below.

However, it is difficult to define the individuals who are at risk. Certainly, the typical patient with osteoporosis is a woman who had an early menopause (either natural or surgically induced), perhaps a late menarche, a poor diet in terms of calcium intake, who abuses tobacco and alcohol and has a positive family history. She may well be too thin.

### 9.14  Is back pain a common sign of osteoporosis?

Unless osteoporosis results in a fractured vertebral body, back pain is virtually never caused by osteoporosis itself. Regardless of whether there is (or is not) osteoporosis present, the primary cause of back pain must be sought. Osteoporosis is a silent epidemic: most patients with osteoporosis are asymptomatic. The epidemic only manifests itself with fractures of the femoral neck or vertebral bodies years too late for treatment. The only symptoms of osteoporosis in the spine are those related to deteriorating posture or height but pain itself virtually never occurs until too late.

### 9.15  What laboratory investigations are appropriate?

If a spinal radiograph reveals osteoporosis then it has to be accepted that this test was performed much too late. For this reason we have to rely on bone densitometry. One single test is often unhelpful and therefore a second test is carried out 12 months later in order to determine not only the state of the bone but the rate of loss of bone. However, all this means an enormous financial outlay and society is perhaps not yet prepared to embark on such a programme.

## 9.16 What are the general principles for preventing osteoporosis?

Bone mineral content peak is reached in the third decade and thereafter there is a slow loss until the menopause when the rate of loss becomes more rapid. Clearly, everything that can be done to produce the highest peak (good exercise, dietary calcium, etc.) and then prevent rapid loss is appropriate. To prevent rapid loss individuals must avoid smoking, drink only moderately, have a high calcium intake and, above all, exercise on a continuing basis.

The main difficulty relates to the timing of the menopause. Obviously, all women who have a surgically induced menopause (bilateral oöphorectomy) or a naturally occurring early menopause must be offered the benefit of hormone replacement therapy (HRT) unless contraindicated.

Contraindications for HRT are few. A strong history of deep vein thromboses with pulmonary emboli is a clear contraindication. Breast cancer or a very strong family history of breast cancer is also a contraindication. Otherwise there are few reasons why an individual should not be given HRT.

Epidemiological studies reveal that death from coronary heart disease and cardiovascular accidents is greatly reduced in HRT takers compared with a control population. Although breast cancer is minimally more prevalent in HRT users, the benefits in terms of population studies greatly outweigh the risk in terms of the few additional cases of breast cancer. Uterine carcinoma can be prevented with the appropriate use of progestogens at the end of the cycle in those with an intact uterus.

## 9.17 How should established osteoporosis be treated?

HRT is still the treatment of choice even in those with established disease. There is no reason why women, even 10 years after their menopause, should not be given HRT. However, it may be appropriate to give additional therapy such as a bisphosphonate in conjunction with calcium. Disodium etidronate has now been licensed for use for the treatment of established osteoporosis. It is given on a sequential basis over a 2-week period followed by 11 weeks on calcium supplements alone followed again by the bisphosphonate. It is currently recommended for use for only 3 years. There are still some concerns as to whether long-term use will translate into *both* quantitative and qualitative improvements. From studies of sodium fluoride, for example, bone densitometry increases dramatically but the *quality* of bone is such that fractures are more, not less, prevalent.

The patient should be encouraged to follow a healthy diet with adequate calcium and sufficient exercise to maintain the skeleton. Of course, smoking and alcohol excess should be avoided.

## INFECTIVE ARTHROPATHIES

### 9.18  What are the common infective arthropathies?

In the UK, the commonest infective arthropathies relate to rubella and other viral entities. However, in immunocompromised individuals or the very old and the young, staphylococcal and streptococcal septic joint disease also occurs.

In general practice, viral infection is much more common than bacterial infection. Viral infection is more likely to be associated with relatively widespread arthralgias and myalgias and a polyarthritis rather than a mono- or oligoarthropathy. In addition, there may well be contact with viral illness within the family. The most common situation would be a young woman presenting with arthralgias and a polyarthritis having had contact with a child who had rubella or some other infection (e.g. parvovirus). In addition, rubella vaccination can result in a widespread synovitis.

### 9.19  What is the management of infective synovitis?

If a bacterial infection is suspected, immediate referral to hospital is required.

First, the nature of the organism should be defined. However, even before the answer to this important question is established antibiotics can be given but only after adequate cultures and synovial fluid aspiration have been performed. Then, if the wrong antibiotic has been selected, the choice would be modified when the laboratory results become available. The common causes, in general practice, of infective synovitis are probably viral, in which case no antibiotic is appropriate; however, in the casualty department or emergency room, staphylococcal arthritis, streptococcal arthritis and even tubercular or fungal arthritis would certainly be expected to be seen. The choice of antibiotic should be discussed with the bacteriology department or public health laboratories. In general, the infected joint should be aspirated once or even daily for a few days if the joint does not settle quickly. Open surgical drainage is very rarely indicated. For example, in a septic hip or sacroiliac joint, open drainage might be required, particularly in a young patient. Depending on the nature of the infection and the type of patient, antibiotics may need to be given for anywhere from 10 days up to 6 weeks, or even longer. Special difficulties arise when a prosthesis becomes infected. Frequently this has to be removed but occasionally long-term antibiotic administration over months may allow the patient to continue with the prosthesis.

### 9.20  How common are other forms of synovitis?

We see, very rarely, patients with infiltrative or deposition synovitis relating to leukaemic infiltration or amyloid deposition. The rheumatologist may well be caught out by such unusual phenomena.

### 9.21  What other disorders may be seen by the GP?

Systemic lupus erythematosus (SLE) is a relatively rare condition. An average GP, for example, may have 10–20 patients with RA, while there may be no cases of SLE. In essence, SLE is a multi-system disorder associated with a positive antinuclear antibody (ANA) and no better diagnosis. For example, a patient with chronic sepsis may develop multisystem disease and an ANA (i.e. antinuclear factor) but in such a situation the diagnosis could be, for example, subacute bacterial endocarditis. If such primary disorders are excluded then one is left with the probability that SLE is the diagnosis. Patients usually present with arthralgia, skin rash, pleurisy or involvement of kidneys, bone marrow and other extra-articular sites. The important point to make about SLE is that the majority of patients with this diagnostic label may not have SLE and, secondly, even those who have it tend to fare well. Severe intractable SLE with multisystem disease is a rare occurrence.

Even rarer are other rheumatological conditions that include polyarteritis nodosa, progressive systemic sclerosis, Wegener's granulomatosis, etc. The interested reader is referred to other texts.

# 10. Paediatric rheumatology

It is a truism that children are not merely little adults and this is particularly true in paediatric rheumatology. There are numerous adult disorders that do not occur in childhood and likewise paediatric diseases that effectively are never seen in adults. The demarcation is arbitrarily taken to be the age of 16 years. Perhaps the most important point is that children grow up into adults and GPs, of course, look after the entire family. It is thus of paramount importance that all of us have familiarity with some of the more common childhood disorders as discussed in this chapter.

## 10.1 How should the common disorders seen in children be approached ?

Although children are not simply small adults, they share with their older counterparts the fact that the common cause of musculoskeletal problems is juxta- and extra-articular rather than articular disease itself. There are numerous painful problems that children develop, which are usually traumatic in origin and self-limiting. For most children, reassurance is more useful than blood tests and radiographic examinations. The exception, of course, is the child with obvious joint swelling, obvious joint dysfunction and those with multisystem disease (i.e. rash, malaise, arthralgias, myalgias, etc.).

In general, children do not develop back pain even when suffering from one of the spondylarthritides. Typically, juvenile AS, for example, presents with a swollen knee or a limp rather than back discomfort.

Table 10.1 summarizes the main features of the juvenile chronic polyarthropathies, and Table 10.2 provides a simple classification.

**Table 10.1** Summary of the main features of juvenile chronic polyarthropathy[1,2]

| Type of onset | Age of onset (years) | Sex ratio | Joint distribution | Serology | Extra-articular disease | Prognosis |
|---|---|---|---|---|---|---|
| Systemic | Young > old | M = F | Any | RF negative | Fever, rash, lymphadenopathy | Usually good, 20% develop polyarthritis, hip involvement |
| Oligoarticular (1) | 10–16 | M > F | Large, hips, sacroiliacs | ANA negative RF negative, B27 positive (75%) | Acute iritis (10%) | Some patients develop ankylosing spondylitis |
| Oligoarticular (2) | 3–5 | F > M | Large | ANA positive (60%) | Chronic iritis | |
| Polyarticular | 10–16 | F > M | Any | RF positive (90%) | Rheumatoid | >50% develop severe arthritis (adult-like disease) |

[1]ANA = antinuclear antibody.
[2]RF = rheumatoid factor.

**Table 10.2** Summary of the modern classification of juvenile chronic arthritis (i.e. persistence > 6 weeks)

1. Acute onset systemic disease (Still's disease)

2. Oligoarticular disease:
   (a) Persistent pauciarticular seronegative arthropathy
   (b) Evolution to seronegative polyarthropathy
   (c) Juvenile onset spondylarthropathy
       (i) Primary ankylosing spondylitis
       (ii) Psoriatic spondylarthropathy
       (iii) Enteropathic spondylarthropathy

3. Seropositive polyarthritis (rheumatoid arthritis)

## 10.2 What is the probable cause of persistent joint swelling?

Children with chronic arthritis (i.e. persistence of joint swelling for 6 weeks or more) have one of several subsets. Systemic onset disease is seen primarily in children between the ages of 2 and 5 years but can occur at any age. This is the subset sometimes called 'Still's disease'. The child is systemically unwell with fever, evanescent rash and a varying degree of joint swelling. In addition, children who present with adult-like seropositive polyarthritis of the rheumatoid type while the majority have an oligo-arthritis, which may evolve into the polyarthritis group or into the juvenile AS. The latter consists predominantly of boys in the teenage years.

## 10.3 When should rheumatic fever be suspected?

Rheumatic fever is exceptionally rare in the UK. There has been a recrudescence of rheumatic fever in children in pockets of middle-class America and it is therefore important that we keep aware of this possibility. Rheumatic fever should be considered in the differential diagnosis of acute systemic onset juvenile arthritis or Still's disease and also must be considered in young children presenting with fevers, malaise and indeed leukaemia.

In general, in children, the old dogma regarding rheumatic fever as 'licking the joints and biting the heart' remains true. In adults, by contrast, post-streptococcal arthritis occurs — reminding us that, in adults, rheumatic fever 'bites the joints and licks the heart'. In fact, we usually see just the joint component in adults.

## 10.4 Does Reiter's syndrome occur in children?

For reasons that are not clearly understood, Reiter's syndrome is exceptionally rare in childhood. For example, in an epidemic of *Shigella flexneri* or one of the other enteropathic organisms that cause reactive arthritis so frequently in adults, children appear to stay healthy in spite of having developed the dysenteric disease. Why children are protected from post-bowel infection reactive arthritis remains unknown. Almost certainly, if we could understand this issue, we would learn much about reactive arthritis in general. The other form of Reiter's disease is sexually acquired reactive arthropathy and naturally, in young children, this is not a problem but it is seen in teenagers — albeit rarely.

## 10.5 Does infectious arthritis occur in children? How should it be managed?

In general, children appear less likely to develop frank arthritis in association with those viral disorders that cause arthropathy in adults. Clearly, children are more likely to develop rubella than are adults and yet rubella arthritis occurs much more readily in the older individual. However, children are at particular risk for staphylococcal arthritis in their early months and years of life. Such infection can affect any large joint, the sacroiliac joint or the spine — giving a staphylococcal discitis, for example. Although the most common age of onset is below 3 years, the occasional teenager presents with an infected discitis. This is something of an emergency and the infective organism should be identified as rapidly as possible so that the correct antibiotic is selected. Where possible, the joint will be drained. For example, a septic hip must be drained rapidly both to provide the nature of the organism and also to decompress the joint. Blood cultures will also be carried out. Antibiotic therapy may be required for 6–12 weeks before the infection is eradicated.

### 10.6  What is the relevance of juvenile osteochondroses?

There are a group of conditions that occur in childhood that relate to pathology at the epiphyses of vertebral bodies, femoral head (Perthes' disease), the navicular bone (Kohler's disease), Kienbock's disease of the lunate and elsewhere. Osgood-Schlatter disease is probably unrelated and presents as pain at the epiphyses of the tibial tubercle.

In large part, these problems are chance radiological findings. However, they may cause a varying degree of symptoms. The prognosis is excellent and usually settles with little medical intervention. For those with more persistent symptoms, orthopaedic surgeons with an interest in such childhood pathology should be referred to.

### 10.7  What points should be stressed about chondromalacia patellae? What is the treatment of choice?

Chondromalacia patellae is an over-diagnosed problem. The term refers to a roughening of the surface between the patella and femoral compartment and, in adults, may be equally labelled as 'patellofemoral osteoarthropathy'. Specifically, the child (or adult) complains of knee pain, particularly on walking down rather than going upstairs. Likewise, athletic activity can bring on the pain. The reason for the pain being worse on walking downstairs is that the quadriceps relaxes, the patella touches the femur and then, on sudden knee extension, the patella runs along the femur recreating the pain. Exercise is the treatment of choice and as the quadriceps musculature is built up, first without and then with weights, the patella is lifted off the femoral compartment and symptoms tend to decrease. Occasionally, an intra-articular corticosteroid injection into the knee will help.

## 10.8  When should malignancy be suspected?

In a child who presents with anaemia, weight loss and anorexia and systemically looks unwell one must think of malignancy — typically a leukaemia in a young child. The other malignancies that are seen in children that can present with musculoskeletal pain relate to osteogenic sarcomas and other rare bone and soft-tissue malignancies. Back pain is exceptionally rare in childhood and if a child presents with back pain and particularly with spinal muscle spasm there should always be a high index of suspicion regarding the possibility of a myosarcoma, fibrosarcoma or other unusual pathology. A straight spinal radiograph may show bone erosion and of course we would follow on with CT, MRI and other studies.

## 10.9  What do we mean by Still's disease?

Childhood inflammatory arthritis includes many different subsets. One of the best known was that originally described by Still. He reported on a group of children, mostly between the ages of 2 and 5 years who had acute illness with systemic features, fever and some joint pains. This became known as Still's disease or, more recently, as acute systemic onset inflammatory arthritis. Interestingly, adults too may develop a comparable entity, although this is relatively unusual.

## 10.10  What are the different forms of chronic juvenile arthritis? How is it managed?

There are several different unrelated forms of chronic juvenile arthritis ranging from the acute systemic onset subset (Still's disease) to seropositive polyarthropathy at the other end of the spectrum. These two disorders are entirely unrelated, the latter mirroring that seen in seropositive RA in adults, while the former condition only rarely has an adult counterpart. In fact, it is now recognized that a few adults have a similar type of disease with fever, malaise, weight loss and varying degree of arthropathy. In childhood, the systemic onset disorder tends to occur during the first 2 or 3 years, while the seropositive disease is predominantly a disorder of teenage girls.

Juvenile psoriatic arthropathy is an entirely separate entity mirroring the adult counterpart; juvenile onset AS also occurs predominantly in teenage boys. This typically presents with a limp and knee or hip pain rather than with spinal symptoms.

Somewhere in the middle of the spectrum is a group of conditions lumped together as a seronegative oligoarticular arthropathy that may finally evolve into AS on the one hand or seropositive polyarthropathy disease on the other. However, the majority continue with a seronegative oligo- or sometimes polyarthropathy.

As with adults, the precise aetiological factors are not understood in spite of knowing something of the genetic associations. In terms of management the main philosophy is that of a multidisciplinary approach with paediatrician, rheumatologist, physiotherapist, hydrotherapist, arthritis nurse, orthopaedic surgeon and, if necessary, child psychologist, family counsellor and other individuals.

### 10.11  What is hypermobility syndrome?

Some 10% of school children have joints that may be considered hypermobile compared with the general population. Not all of these are symptomatic but when epidemiological studies have addressed the problem it has become apparent that among those children with joint and muscle pains, more have hypermobility than one would expect by chance alone.

Hypermobile children may be recognized if they can bend to the floor with knees straight and place their palms on the ground, or have hyperextension at the elbow greater than 5 degrees, hyperextensibility at the knee with extension of over 5 degrees, the ability to touch the volar surface of their forearm with their thumb and hyperextensibility of the digits that can reach 75–90 degrees rather than the more normal 30–40 degrees. Not all these features may be present but in such children (or adults) symptoms may be generalized or relate to certain groups of muscles and joints.

The most common area of concern relates to the knees, hips

and shoulders — the lower limb joints being particularly problematic in teenage children who are active with sporting activities. They may well find that running becomes a major problem. Unfortunately, children with hyperextensibility are sometimes encouraged to take up ballet dancing and it is these very individuals who are at risk of damage and professional frustration.

## 10.12 How is it treated?

The first and most important aspect relates to strong reassurance that the patient (child or adult) does not have a sinister underlying disease and that symptoms usually decrease rather than increase. Secondly, it is worth stressing that this problem is well recognized and commonly mismanaged. For example, in the past many such children were said to have 'growing pains', while others were thought to be malingering and trying to avoid school sporting activities for reasons other than medical ones.

In general, apart from this reassurance, treatment is directed towards enhancing the musculature. If the knees are primarily affected then quadriceps exercises, at first without and then with weights, would be appropriate. With hip involvement, attention to the lumbar musculature with isometric flexion exercises is of paramount importance. The best activity is, without doubt, swimming, which allows the musculature to be strengthened without any further damage to the underlying joint and joint capsules.

## 10.13 Should a child with musculoskeletal disorders be referred to a paediatrician or a rheumatologist?

The ideal situation is a combined clinic with a paediatrician and rheumatologist as we have at The Royal National Hospital for Rheumatic Diseases in Bath. This is unusual and, in general, paediatricians would see children, referring those with a clearly defined complicated arthropathy to a rheumatologist. It also depends on the age. It would seem natural not to send a child of 12 years or more with a swollen knee, ankle or polyarthritis to a paediatrician since a rheumatologist would be more familiar with this type of problem than his or her paediatric counterpart.

## 10.14  When should a child be referred?

I would recommend referral at any time if the parents are anxious or if the GP does not feel confident in reassuring the parents and child. I would never consider that a child (or for that matter, adult) has been referred too early. Clearly, any child with chronic arthritis should be referred and I would also expect to see children with, for example, multiple joint pains of unclear aetiology. We frequently find that such children, who may have a hypermobility syndrome with inevitable joint pains, cause great concern for the parents.

Parents will always be anxious about a child with a rheumatological problem and they can usually be reassured that the situation will be self-limiting or even if persistent, very mild. Most childhood aches and pains settle quite simply and even chronic arthritis carries a fairly good prognosis.

## 10.15  How should trauma be managed?

Any child presenting with, for example, a swollen knee may admit to a previous traumatic episode and it is easy to assume cause and effect. Clearly, it is of importance to establish precisely the nature of the trauma and determine whether it really was sufficient to cause the problem. In general, any traumatic joint lesion will settle within 2 or 3 days whereas an inflammatory problem will persist.

# 11. Approaches to treatment

Our first approach to the treatment of systemic or long-term diseases such as RA and OA must be the education of the patient. He or she must learn about the condition and what to expect. The role of the GP and the rheumatologist must be explained. The place for investigations, diet, exercise, rest, physiotherapy, occupational therapy, surgery and drug management must be understood. Where possible, family members should be present at the consultation to support what has been said. This chapter concentrates on the drug treatments available, and the principles of long-term patient care.

## DRUG TREATMENT

This section deals with simple analgesics, NSAIDs and disease-modifying agents. Inevitably the major issue is one of safety and efficacy. Regrettably, we do not yet have an ideal agent and so the GP and rheumatologist must always weigh up the potential benefit and the potential risks. The principles of corticosteroid injection are also outlined.

### 11.1 What are the general principles of drug treatment?

First, I try to start with local therapy if possible. In general, simple analgesics are safer than non-steroidal agents, and NSAIDs are safer than systemic corticosteroids. For patients with more generalized inflammatory disease (such as RA) early use of a disease-modifying agent (e.g. methotrexate in conjunction with an NSAID) is appropriate.

SIMPLE ANALGESICS

## 11.2 What straightforward analgesics are of use in the management of rheumatological conditions?

Paracetamol (acetaminophen in the USA) is certainly the simplest and is probably the most used. Thereafter, many patients favour co-proxamol (a mixture of dextropropoxyphene hydrochloride 32.5 mg and paracetamol 325 mg) and a variety of other paracetamol mixtures. For example, co-codamol (containing codeine phosphate 8 mg and paracetamol 500 mg) and co-dydramol (dihydrocodeine tartrate 10 mg and paracetamol 500 mg) are popular among many patients with arthritis. In my experience, the most common of all these is co-proxamol, which has replaced distalgesic (no longer available on the NHS). These agents are well-tolerated and deal with the patient's greatest concern — pain. Clearly, the GP must be aware of what is contained in these poly-pharmacy analgesics. For example, co-codaprin contains aspirin and should therefore be avoided in children and in adults intolerant of aspirin or in those receiving aspirin or a NSAID separately.

## 11.3 What other analgesics are available?

There are numerous other analgesics such as nefopam hydrochloride and other compound analgesic preparations with various mixtures of aspirin, paracetamol and codeine — none of which are now generally recommended.

Single-ingredient preparations should generally be prescribed in preference to the compound analgesics because the compounds rarely have any advantage and certainly complicate the treatment of overdose. Nevertheless, there is a suggestion that agents such as dextropropoxyphene-paracetamol are more 'efficacious' than paracetamol or dextropropoxyphene alone. However, hard scientific data are few. It is probable, at least, that dextropropoxyphene has some CNS stimulatory effect, which adds to its popularity.

Patients should be warned when compound analgesics contain paracetamol so that they can avoid other paracetamol-containing preparations, and the potential for inadvertent overdose with potential hepatotoxicity.

## 11.4 What is the role of the opiates?

In rheumatological practice, opioid analgesics should almost always be avoided and, in general, if pethidine, morphine, buprenorphine, dextramoramide, dextropropoxyphene, pentazocine or other agents are required, consultation with a rheumatologist would be appropriate. It may well be that the entire problem needs to be reviewed and a different approach to analgesia taken in such patients.

## 11.5 Is there a 'rule of thumb' for the use of simple analgesics?

Virtually all rheumatological conditions are painful and what follows relates to the problems that may present to the primary physician.

Always start with paracetamol. If that fails, consider the relative advantages of an NSAID or a combination agent such as co-proxamol (dextropropoxyphene 32.5 mg/paracetamol 325 mg). In essence, the latter may be better tolerated than the former — particularly in older patients. The major difference relates to overdose. It is very difficult to do much damage when overdosing on an NSAID but any paracetamol-containing agent can be lethal in such a situation.

If the analgesic has little effect the agent should be stopped and a new approach taken. If the patient continues to require analgesia after 3 or 4 weeks, again a new approach should be considered. As mentioned several times elsewhere in this text, if local pain appears to be the problem then local therapy should be considered.

## NSAIDS

## 11.6 What is the place of the NSAIDs in the treatment of rheumatological conditions?

By definition, NSAIDs should only be used where there is inflammation. For many years it was thought that degenerative arthropathy (OA, osteoarthrosis) was purely mechanical in nature but we now recognize that many of the symptoms relate to inflammatory episodes. These can result from secondary inflammation of the synovium related to cartilage and bone debris or crystals released from cartilage and other mechanisms.

NSAIDs are indicated in rheumatoid disease, osteoarthropathy, AS and 'acute' musculoskeletal disorders. NSAIDs are frequently more efficacious than analgesics alone. Nevertheless, in an ideal situation, an analgesic should be used alone if possible given that such an agent is better tolerated in the long term.

For patients with generalized inflammatory disease such as RA or polyarticular psoriaic arthropathy, NSAIDs are a must. Exceptions to this would be the patient with RA who is well-controlled on, for example, methotrexate, and may get by with the occasional use of a simple analgesic and not require an NSAID. Also, in individuals who have had NSAID toxicity in the past, low-dose prednisolone may be the safer option.

### 11.7 There are something over 20 NSAIDs on the market at the moment. Which one should a GP pick for any particular problem?

The GP should be familiar with two or three (or at the most four) non-steroidal agents. In general, the efficacy is much the same but certain people tolerate one better than another. My approach is to go with the once-a-day agent. This may be a slow-release preparation of an agent with a short half-life, or a drug with a long half-life such as an oxicam. Once-a-day drugs provide the best patient compliance and therefore the best efficacy. By contrast, an older woman, for example, who has had a lot of problems with many agents, may be given the weakest NSAID, which almost certainly would be ibuprofen with a short half-life. This needs to be taken three or four times a day. You may wish to give her that in a low dose hoping she will forget once or twice and therefore she will be less at risk from side-effects. Alternatives for patients with a poor gastrointestinal history include nabumetone or the newer slow-release ibuprofen preparations.

In summary, the following points should be considered by the GP when choosing which NSAID to prescribe:

• *Experience in the marketplace.* The longer a drug has been available, the better its toxicity profile is known, making it suitable for at-risk patients. For example, indomethacin is one of the oldest, most respected NSAIDs and is highly efficacious; other drugs include aspirin, low-dose ibuprofen or nabumetone.

- *Tolerability versus efficacy.* The safer the drug, the less efficacious. For example, ibuprofen is the one of safest drug but probably the least efficacious NSAID. Drugs with a short half-life require multiple dosing and may lead to poor compliance, whereas long half-life agents and slow-release agents can be given once per day, which improves compliance and therefore the risk of side-effects.
- *Route of administration.* In the UK, we prefer the oral route. By contrast, some continental Europeans like the per-rectal route! Although local stomach irritation is less, most toxicity relates to the systemic effect, and therefore there is no major advantage for the non-oral approach. Intramuscular preparations may be used postoperatively or in the 'emergency' situation.
- *Side-effect/patient group.* NSAIDs are most risky for the old, for those with a positive history of gastrointestinal bleeds or ulcers, or for those on corticosteroids, for those who smoke or abuse alcohol, for those on anticoagulants. Some drug side-effects that are more common in certain groups, e.g. indomethacin is more likely to cause headaches in older women, so the class of NSAID can be changed to avoid certain side-effects.

These factors are explored in more detail under the following headings.

## Experience of use

### 11.8 Which of the NSAIDs do we have the most experience of?

*Aspirin and salicylates*

Aspirin is still appropriately recognized as a powerful cost-effective agent, which, if well tolerated, causes few problems long term. Historically, there have been difficulties with compliance but this has been resolved with the newer aspirins that need only be taken once or twice daily, although these new aspirins tend to be more expensive and so less cost-effective. Certainly, no new NSAID is more efficacious than aspirin though most are better tolerated than regular soluble aspirin on its own.

Aspirin is also available in paracetamol combinations (e.g. benorylate) but there are no data supporting the combination as being more efficacious than aspirin alone with the addition of paracetamol prn. One advantage, however, is the fact that it is a liquid and many individuals prefer this over tablet forms of medication. The aspirin-paracetamol mixture of 10 ml is made up of 2.3 g aspirin and 1940 mg paracetamol. The usual dose is 10 ml daily in rheumatoid disease. The price of the aspirin-paracetamol preparation is roughly £0.60 per day compared with some £0.05 for regular dispersible aspirin. Other newer salicylate preparations are also available, such as choline magnesium trisalicylate and sodium salicylate. The side-effects relate to gastrointestinal toxicity and aspirin-associated tinnitus.

*Ibuprofen*

Ibuprofen was introduced in the late 1960s and has been available for almost 25 years. Initially it was introduced at a low dose of 200 mg thrice daily and although this was associated with an almost placebo-like action, it was well tolerated! Since then the dose has steadily increased and it is now common to give 2400 mg of ibuprofen or even more! Certainly, these large doses of ibuprofen are less well tolerated than the very low doses but nevertheless the toxicity profile is certainly a major selling point. Indeed, over the counter sales are now permitted at a dose of up to 1200 mg daily, although this is certainly not sufficient for most patients with rheumatoid disease. Nevertheless, it is a relatively safe analgesic when compared with paracetamol with the added advantage of an anti-inflammatory effect. Recently sustained-release and retard preparations have been made available. One point of concern, however, is that patients may be on prescribed ibuprofen by their GP and unknowingly take additional over-the-counter (OTC) ibuprofen such as 'Nurofen' unaware that both contain the same active ingredient. Moreover, the OTC preparation is much more expensive than the prescribed generic preparation.

*Indomethacin*

For over 20 years, indomethacin has been considered the drug of choice for gout and seronegative spondylarthritides where it appears to have a particularly beneficial effect on this enthesopathic group of disorders. Indomethacin is perceived to be the most efficacious agent and this is probably a justified claim; it is described as the 'gold standard' by which other NSAIDs are judged. Virtually every new NSAID is tested against indomethacin for that very reason. Within the last 3 years we have carried out a study of over 2000 patients with AS, in a transnational investigation, and found, again, that indomethacin was the favoured agent both in terms of numbers taking the drug and, more importantly, in those still taking the drug after a 2-year period.

The availability of 25 and 50 mg capsules and a 75 mg slow-release preparation, together with a suppository form of 100 mg, allows for three or four times per day medication or once a day usage.

However, the most important advantage is that the toxicity profile is very well recognized. The major problems with the drug relate to gastrointestinal toxicity and central nervous system side-effects. The former problem is shared with most of the NSAIDs drugs if not all of them to a varying degree. However, the CNS toxicity appears to be a problem particularly in older women and can be partly overcome by dosing at night. There is less of a problem using acemetacin, which is related to indomethacin and may have its advantages of efficacy without the CNS disadvantages.

## 11.9 Should any precautions be taken against unexpected complications with the newer preparations?

In general, any new agent should be used with caution. In essence, a new drug appearing on the market has been carefully studied in some 2000 individuals at the most. Clearly, an unusual side-effect that occurs in one individual in every 10 000 may have been missed. By contrast, most of the major NSAIDs that have been available for at least 1–2 years have been prescribed to 100 000 patients or more. As post-marketing surveillance becomes more sophisticated, we can quickly get the feel for 'unexpected' events once the drug has been in the marketplace for a year or more. Thus, to avoid 'unexpected' complications, select a drug that has been available for at least 1 or 2 years and then, at least, any of the rarer side-effects can be anticipated.

Another note of caution with relatively new agents is that the dose range has still not been adequately defined in different age groups. If a relatively new agent is required, a healthy middle-aged or younger individual rather than an octogenarian should be selected to 'experiment with'.

## 11.10 What are the simple 'rules-of-thumb' to be observed in the use of NSAIDs?

1. Only use an NSAID if a simple analgesic fails.
2. When possible, treat local problems with local therapy (e.g. intralesional corticosteroid).
3. Try to avoid NSAIDs in patients at risk (e.g. older women with a past history of NSAID-related toxicity).
4. If giving an NSAID to someone at particular risk, try to use a low-dose short half-life agent for a short period. An example of such a drug would be ibuprofen 400 mg bid for 2 weeks.
5. In young, otherwise healthy individuals with an inflammatory disease, once-a-day preparations are often preferable given better compliance and greater disease control. Examples of once-a-day NSAIDs include indomethacin 75 mg slow-release (Indomax 75), diclofenac 100 mg slow-release (Voltarol Retard), flurbiprofen 200 mg slow-release (Froben SR), piroxicam 20 mg each night, tenoxicam 20 mg and other agents.
6. If one class of agent causes toxicity try another agent, which may have a different profile of side-effects and therefore be better suited to a given individual. For example, if indomethacin results in side-effects, one could try diclofenec — or *vice versa*.
7. If gastrointestinal toxicity is a concern, consider nabumetone, or another drug with a good track record or decide whether to give prophylaxis with an $H_2$-antagonist (e.g. ranitidine) or misoprostol.

### Tolerance versus efficacy

## 11.11 Is there a trade-off between efficacy and tolerability?

Yes, in part. There is no doubt that, in the past, the powerful NSAIDs such as indomethacin and the weaker ones such as ibuprofen were considered to be the two ends of the spectrum. However, perhaps more important than relative 'strength' is compliance. Once-a-day drugs with a long half-life, such as piroxicam, result in better compliance than short half-life agents such as ibuprofen. Inevitably, with a multiple-dosing schedule the patient may forget to take the drug once or twice per day. So the outcome is less efficacy and certainly more tolerability.

## 11.12 Does cyclo-oxygenase inhibiting activity affect efficacy?

In fact, it makes little difference. For example, flurbiprofen, a fluorinated ibuprofen is a strong cyclo-oxygenase inhibitor and is not obviously more or less efficacious than azapropazone, a drug that is less 'strong' in terms of prostaglandin synthesis inhibition. One reason for this may be that NSAIDs work in a variety of different ways that include cyclo-oxygenase inhibition and the capacity to alter monocyte cell activity and function.

## 11.13 Are short half-life NSAIDs better tolerated than long half-life agents?

In essence there is little evidence that drugs with a short half-life (e.g. ibuprofen) are better tolerated than those with a long half-life (e.g. the oxicams). Given that a drug with a long half-life can be prescribed once a day and a drug with a short half-life three or four times per day, these data translate into good or bad compliance and, as discussed above, the apparent better safety profile with the short-acting half-life drugs.

For most of the modern NSAIDs, accumulation of the long half-life drugs is not a real problem, even in the aged population. Drugs with a middle-range half-life (e.g. naproxen, indomethacin, diclofenac) are not obviously different from the agents at the two extremes.

## 11.14 Are slow-release preparations better tolerated than divided doses of the regular compound?

There is no evidence that slow-release preparations of indomethacin, ketoprofen, flurbiprofen, ibuprofen, naproxen or other agents are better tolerated than the same drug in the conventional form. Indeed, the reverse may be so — not because the drug is more toxic in the 'retard' preparation but simply because compliance is better and therefore more drug is ingested and so more likely to cause side-effects.

In general, studies have suggested that if a tablet is required to be taken once daily in arthritis, the compliance is some 90% whereas for twice-a-day preparations the compliance falls to 80% and for thrice daily preparations there is a further fall to 70%. Drugs taken qds reveal a compliance that is no better than 65%.

Our understanding of chronobiology suggests that, in general, the medication should be given in the evening since this has a beneficial effect on early morning stiffness and any side-effects are 'missed' during the night when the patient is unaware of a small amount of gastrointestinal discomfort or headaches, for example. One study clearly showed that indomethacin 75 mg as a slow-release preparation was better tolerated overall and more efficacious when given at night than in the morning or at midday. Although this has not been studied with other agents, it is likely to be true for them as well.

## Routes of administration

### 11.15 What are the advantages and disadvantages of the various routes of administration?

Before slow-release preparations by mouth became available, the suppository had the added advantage of steady absorption during the night with the relief of morning stiffness. Another advantage is that gastrointestinal tract irritation is less but, because many of the side-effects relate to circulating drug (i.e. a systemic effect) rather than direct contact of the agent on the gastric mucosa, this is something of a theoretical rather than a practical advantage. A major disadvantage of the suppository approach is that the agent may be poorly absorbed or lost prior to absorption. Moreover, anal irritation may occur. Also, many patients, especially in the UK, refuse to use suppositories. Therefore, now with the enteric coated/slow-release/sustained-release preparations, there are fewer advantages to using suppositories.

Intramuscular preparations are available for many of the NSAIDs and their advantage is speed of onset. For example, in patients with renal colic, intramuscular diclofenac or other NSAID is helpful. Also, post-operative analgesia with an injectable NSAID is appropriate since medicine by mouth would not be possible in such a situation.

Transcutaneous NSAIDs are now available for several preparations including ibuprofen, diclofenac, ketoprofen and felbinac (the active ingredient of fenbufen). The advantage of transcutaneous preparations is local application of the drug for local pathology and the patient has control over the use of the medication. However, the topical NSAIDs are expensive and are almost certainly less efficacious than a local steroid injection. Secondly, there are no data supporting their use in comparison to the rubifacients that are available at 10–15% of the price. Although the pharmaceutical industry has shown that the non-steroidal preparation is more efficacious than placebo, the appropriate studies against cheaper preparations have not been carried out.

Sublingual piroxicam ('Melt') suits individuals who dislike taking tablets. Although it has not been studied in comparison to 20 mg piroxicam tablets, intuitively one would anticipate that there could be less gastrointestinal toxicity in as much as the agent is not in direct contact with the gastric lining. However, the systemic side-effect profile would be the same.

## Side-effects/patient group

### 11.16 What are the main facts regarding NSAID-induced bleeding?

The important points to remember with NSAID-induced gastropathy may be summarized as follows:

1. In endoscopic studies it has been shown that some 20% of individuals on NSAIDs have erosions or small ulcers at any one time.
2. If the same group of individuals are re-endoscoped 6 weeks later some 20% are again found with endoscopic change but many of the old lesions have healed and the 20% figure now includes new patients who were asymptomatic some weeks earlier. If the procedure is repeated 6 weeks later a different 20% population will be found to have endoscopic change!
3. There is almost no relationship between endoscopic evidence of damage and symptoms reported by the patient.
4. It is very difficult to recognize which patient is destined to develop a massive and potentially fatal gastrointestinal bleed, apart from those featured in the at-risk list given below.
5. There are two major goals relating to NSAID-induced gastropathy management. The first is to decrease the symptoms that the patient complains of (anorexia, indigestion, nausea, vomiting, abdominal pain, etc.). Secondly, the physician and patient are concerned about the risk of a massive gastrointestinal bleed or perforation and the 10% of such individuals who do not survive following this major medical event.

6. An additional problem related to NSAIDs is that of clinically silent anaemia. The haemoglobin progressively falls because of asymptomatic blood loss. Associated with the anaemia, the patient becomes progressively fatigued and weak.

## 11.17  Who is at risk of GI bleeding?

The specific individuals at risk include the following:

1. Women.
2. Age over 75–80 years.
3. Relatively recent introduction of an NSAID (i.e. within 2–3 months).
4. Those who abuse alcohol.
5. Those who abuse tobacco.
6. Those on corticosteroid therapy.
7. Those with a past history of gastrointestinal bleed or major gastrointestinal discomfort.
8. Those on anticoagulants.
9. In addition, the sick and infirm are inevitably at greater risk than otherwise healthy subjects.

However, anyone is at risk, anytime.

## 11.18  How would the risk of a major gastrointestinal bleed be reduced in such patients?

The major approach is to avoid the use of an NSAID where possible in individuals at risk. For example, many patients with localized pain resulting from a degenerative joint or ligamentous problem could be managed with a simple analgesic, advice about appropriate exercises, local corticosteroid injection or even an NSAID transcutaneous preparation. A few cases of RA can be managed with a disease-modifying agent or even low-dose oral prednisolone (less than 5 mg per day).

For those who do need an NSAID, a short course is always preferable to long-term medication. Frequent review is necessary. Moreover, the lowest possible dose compatible with the patient's well being should be prescribed.

For patients at risk who require long-term NSAID therapy, it may be appropriate to co-prescribe an $H_2$-antagonist or miso-prostol.

## 11.19 How efficacious is misoprostol?

Misoprostol is a prostaglandin analogue. It certainly decreases the incidence of new NSAID-induced erosions and ulcers as assessed by endoscopic evaluation. However, most studies suggest that an NSAID plus misoprostol produces more symptoms than does an NSAID plus placebo. The outstanding question is whether misoprostol reduces the risk of NSAID-induced massive gastrointestinal bleeds and therefore death. The appropriate epidemiological data are now becoming available. The outcome of a major study looking at several thousand subjects suggests that misoprostol at 200µg four times daily decreases the risk of major gastrointestinal side-effects by some 50%Misoprostol and diclofenac are now being marketed in a fused medication known as Arthrotec.

Put simply, the 20% figure at risk of bleeding may be reduced to perhaps 5% by misoprostol but, given that only one individual in a thousand would bleed, can we be sure that the 75% reduction, from 20% to 5%, will have an impact on the one subject per thousand that really concerns us (i.e. the perforation or massive bleed)? The definitive cost/benefit study is needed. We know that misoprostol causes diarrhoea and many cannot tolerate the drug. Secondly, the financial cost may be prohibitive unless data can reveal more precisely at-risk patients who are likely to benefit.

Endoscopic data support misoprostol over the $H_2$-antagonists in terms of the presence of new lesions but $H_2$-antagonists cause virtually no side-effects and deal with the NSAID-induced symptoms more efficiently.

Finally, misoprostol is absolutely contraindicated in women who may be pregnant given that the agent acts as an abortifacient.

## 11.20 What are the side-effects of NSAIDs other than gastrointestinal bleeding?

Side-effects include diarrhoea, dyspepsia, nausea, constipation, abdominal pain, perforation, flatulence, headache and CNS dysfunction, dizziness, skin rashes and, rarely, other events (e.g. renal damage).

## 11.21 Why was phenylbutazone withdrawn from general use?

Phenylbutazone was the drug of choice in seronegative arthritis.

However, it is only available for use among rheumatologists for patients with spondylarthritis or rather, even more specifically, for those with ankylosing spondylitis. Phenylbutazone, for reasons that are not apparent, is as efficacious as indomethacin and may even have an advantage in ankylosing spondylitis — there being patients who only do well on this drug.

In essence, the concern relating to phenylbutazone was that, in older patients, aplastic anaemia occurs in some one in 60 000 individuals. Agranulocytosis is much less common and is idiosyncratic in nature whereas the aplastic anaemia appears to be a dose-related toxic effect. In the past, many older individuals (over 60 years of age) with degenerative arthropathy were given phenylbutazone and clearly in this situation aplastic anaemia is an unacceptable side-effect. However, when used carefully, phenylbutazone is still a fine agent. In younger patients, idiosyncratic agranulocytosis occurs in less than two or three cases per million.

### 11.22 Can some NSAIDs destroy the cartilage in the hip joint while other NSAIDs spare it?

There is much interest focusing on chondroprotection and chondrodestruction. In essence, it is very easy (but misleading) to extrapolate from *in vitro*, *ex vivo* and other laboratory data to the human situation. Numerous studies have been performed with tissue culture and animal experimentation and the conclusion from these studies is that not all non-steroidal agents have exactly the same effect on cartilage. Some have a relatively neutral effect, while others have a somewhat destructive effect. However, at the moment there is no clinical evidence that cartilage is damaged to a significant degree by NSAIDs. There have been some reports of an accelerated cartilage loss in patients receiving NSAIDs, referred to as 'analgesic hip' by some surgeons. However, it must be stressed that since patients taking an analgesic/non-steroidal agent already have joint disease and clearly non-steroidal agents cannot suppress the disease in its entirety, it may well be that those destined to rapid destruction will suffer regardless of whether they are on an NSAID. It is dangerous to suggest that there is a cause and effect relationship. Also, it must be appreciated that the more a damaged joint is used, the more it will deteriorate and it is possible that, in individuals who are satisfied from an analgesic point of view, increased stresses will be met by the joint through increased use, and this in turn could be associated with the accelerated destruction.

In summary, the ideal NSAID does not exist and there is certainly no drug in the 1990s that can prevent cartilage destruction in those with degenerative joint disease.

### 11.23 Why are some NSAIDs recommended for use in children while others are not?

In large part this depends on whether the appropriate studies have been performed and whether, for this reason, a licence has been granted for use in childhood conditions. Almost certainly there is no difference in the risk of different non-steroidal agents in childhood but it makes good clinical sense to use agents that have been 'passed' for use in childhood practice. For example, naproxen can also be used in children with juvenile arthropathy at a dose of 10 mg/kg body weight but should be avoided in those less than 5 years of age. Tolmetin is approved for use in children in a range of 20–25 mg/kg daily in three or four doses. Mefenamic acid is also available for use in children.

### 11.24 Why is aspirin no longer recommended for use in children?

Aspirin is no longer recommended in children under the age of 12 years because of the possible development of Reye's syndrome. However, there are exceptions to this rule, as with every other in medicine. For example, in acute onset systemic Still's disease, aspirin may still be considered the drug of choice but particular care should be taken by the supervising physician in this situation.

### 11.25 What is Reye's syndrome?

Encephalopathy with fatty degeneration of viscera associated with hepatomegaly and raised liver enzymes has been known as Reye's syndrome after Dr Corrie Reye who described the condition in children between 1 and 12 years of age. Hyperglycaemia is frequently a feature in children below the age of 5 years. There is usually an antecedent viral-type illness, most often chicken pox or influenza B. An association with aspirin administration has been reported.

## SECOND-LINE OR DISEASE-MODIFYING DRUGS

### 11.26 What are the important features of second-line agents?

Second-line drugs are variously known as slow-acting agents, disease-modifying drugs, penicillamine-like drugs, remission-inducing drugs and other labels. However, no label is accurate given that: (1) there is no absolute proof that these drugs actually modify the disease; (2) it is difficult to define the term 'slow-acting'; and (3) there is no evidence that NSAIDs actually fail to modify disease. Dealing with the last point first, the only way to prove whether NSAIDs do or do not modify disease is to give 1000 patients with RA, for example, an NSAID and 1000 patients a placebo. I would anticipate that there would be less inflammation and less joint damage in those receiving long-term NSAIDs (clearly, this study would be unethical). The concept of 'slow-acting' is helpful but methotrexate, for example, begins to work in about 3 weeks whereas the other 'slow-acting' drugs usually start to work by 10–14 weeks. Clearly some are slower than others. Next, come the new monoclonal antibodies directed at a variety of relevant molecules and these almost certainly work within days rather than months and yet may well modify disease

Finally, there is a debate as to whether the so-called disease-modifying agents really modify disease. Given that I believe that NSAIDs do, it is almost certain that the disease-modifying agents do, and more so, but few are tolerated for more than a year or so and there is often a disease breakthrough, so it is difficult to prove the point. Moreover, disease 'modification' needs to be defined in terms of symptoms, function, joint deformity and other variables.

### 11.27 What second-line agents are recommended?

My preference is for methotrexate. In the UK, there are still rheumatologists who like to use penicillamine, gold or hydroxy-chloroquine before methotrexate, while others are happier with sulphasalazine. Most of the world literature on this subject suggests that methotrexate is the preferred agent given that more people tolerate methotrexate for longer and efficacy is better. Thus, 12–24 months after embarking on a disease-modifying agent some 50–80% of patients have been withdrawn from penicillamine, gold, sulphasalazine and other drugs. By contrast, the figure for methotrexate is perhaps only 20 or 25%, in part because it is better tolerated and in part because of better efficacy. I therefore begin with this agent and move onto the others only if necessary. From the patient's point of view, methotrexate is an easy first choice. It is easier to take two or three tablets once per week than, for example, four daily (i.e. sulphasalazine).

### 11.28  When should use of more than one disease-modifying agent at the same time be considered?

Very rarely. In general, using more than one potentially toxic drug increases the risk of toxicity while efficacy is only minimally, if at all, increased. This is in marked contrast to the situation in oncology.

### 11.29  At what stage should we consider second-line or disease-modifying agents?

This must depend on the experience of the practitioner. My own approach is to begin methotrexate or one of the other disease-modifying agents immediately I am satisfied that the patient really has seropositive rheumatoid disease. In addition, I would use this agent for any patient with psoriatic arthropathy or reactive arthropathy that does not respond within a few weeks to adequate NSAID therapy, intra-articular corticosteroid injection and sensible advice about exercise, rest and other modalities.

Once I have a good remission with methotrexate at, for example, 7.5 mg weekly, I would reduce the dose to 7.5 mg alternating with 5 mg weekly, followed by 5 mg, followed by 5 mg alternating with 2.5 mg and eventually reach 2.5 mg, for example, to be taken every other week. In general, the disease-modifying drugs must be used in the same way as insulin in that treatment is for life but with a tapering dose if possible. In general, dose changes may be made every 12 or so weeks. If necessary, methotrexate can be given at a dose of up to 20 mg weekly.

### 11.30  What about the use of these agents in women of child-bearing age?

Clearly there are exceptions to the above approach. I would not necessarily want to start a young woman who is anxious to become pregnant with a potentially dangerous drug such as methotrexate. If possible, any disease-modifying agent should be avoided while a decision regarding early pregnancy is made. If there is no alternative to a disease-modifying drug, very low-dose prednisolone (5 mg or less) may, in this situation, be appropriate. However, once it is clear that simple modalities are not working then a disease-modifying drug such as methotrexate must be considered seriously. Often, the dosage can begin to be tapered after 6 months or so and the drug even withdrawn completely for the period during which the patient is pregnant.

### 11.31 What guidelines should the GP follow about stepping in with second-line agents?

Really the decision has to be whether to begin to use a disease-modifying agent or whether to refer the patient to a rheumatologist. If the practitioner is familiar with hydroxychloroquine or sulphasalazine for individuals with milder disease then there is no reason why the drugs should not be introduced. However, if the disease is not mild then I would recommend referral to a rheumatologist for early initiation of, for example, methotrexate therapy. Personally, I would give methotrexate at a low dose even for mild disease.

In either case, I think it very helpful for a rheumatologist to see the patient early on to confirm the diagnosis and agree with a decision about use of a disease-modifying agent. As discussed elsewhere, this is an excellent opportunity for shared care. Patients may be seen once per year by the rheumatologist and for the rest of the time by the GP.

### 11.32 What should the GP be aware of once the patient has been started on a second-line agent?

In the ideal situation, the rheumatologist will give some written instructions both to the patient and to the GP. As the GP becomes involved with one or two disease-modifying agents he or she can follow the instructions recommended by the rheumatologist. In general, the GP will follow the patient on a monthly basis, while the rheumatologist may see the patient once or twice per year. Again, it must be stressed that there should be close contact between the specialist and the GP and this can be by written communication or/and by telephone.

It is of extreme importance that the patient has been educated about the drug. The patient must take responsibility for ensuring that regular blood tests or other investigations are carried out. Likewise, the GP must follow up the results since laboratory abnormalities still occasionally return to the surgery and are filed without the GP, patient or rheumatologist becoming aware of the toxicity that is developing.

Special attention needs to be focused on following specific drugs:

1. *Hydroxychloroquine.* In general this is the safest disease-modifying drug. Patients usually begin with 200 mg twice daily for 3–4 months followed by 200 mg daily. There is some debate as to whether ophthalmic evaluation by the ophthalmologist is necessary. In general, we feel this not to be the case but some would argue that it is a good idea to have an ophthalmic assessment in the unlikely event that the patient continues the drug for more than 4–5 years. Laboratory tests are not indicated apart from those used to assess the clinical outcome (e.g. haemoglobin, plasma viscosity or ESR).

2. *Methotrexate.* This is one of the easier drugs to use. The most important side-effects relate to pulmonary toxicity and therefore the patient must be warned that any shortness of breath or dry cough must immediately be brought to the attention of the physician but in the meantime methotrexate ingestion must be stopped. This can always be reintroduced once the situation is reviewed. Baseline full blood picture, platelet count and liver function tests should be performed and repeated at 2 weeks. I would then repeat this each month for 3 months and then if all is well and the dose maintained at 7.5 mg once per week I would carry out the blood tests every 6 weeks. Clearly, in a patient who has had a bad experience with other drugs in the past, the physician would be more attentive. There is very little correlation between changing liver function tests and meaningful hepatic pathology but, in general, should the tests increase by a factor of three, then the situation should be reviewed — perhaps withdrawing the drug at least *pro tem.* Personally, I do not request a baseline chest radiograph although this has been recommended. However, as

the world of rheumatology becomes more experienced with the use of this drug, some of the older views are disappearing. For instance, rheumatologists virtually never get a liver biopsy at any stage.

3. *Penicillamine.* Monthly full blood picture and platelet count is required together with urinalysis looking for protein and red cells. If more than two ++ of protein appears on a dipstick test then a 24 hour urinary protein should be performed and, if more than 2 g are being excreted, one should consider stopping the drug and perhaps reintroducing it later at a lower level. However, some find even 2.5–3 g protein loss per 24 hours acceptable.

4. *Gold.* The same comments apply to gold as to penicillamine.

5. *Azathioprine and cyclophosphamide.* These drugs are potentially more myelotoxic and for the first month 2-weekly blood tests should be carried out followed by monthly tests indefinitely, keeping a close eye on platelet count, haemoglobin and white cell count.

In general, the GP must be familiar with the small print regarding all of these potentially dangerous drugs. (See Appendix 2 for summary guidelines for monitoring second-line agents.)

### 11.33 What are the major problems that arise when these drugs are prescribed?

Almost certainly the biggest catastrophes follow misprescribing. For example, we still see patients who are given methotrexate 7.5 mg daily rather than weekly, which can be lethal within 2 or 3 weeks. Unfortunately, there are several stages at which a mistake can be made. The rheumatologist may misdictate the letter. The transcriber of the dictation may mistranscribe the instructions, the GP may misread the instructions, the prescription written by the GP may be written incorrectly, the pharmacist may misread the prescription or the patient may be given the wrong dose in spite of the correct prescription having been written and finally the patient may take the wrong dose, misunderstanding the instructions!

Also, when monitoring the patient, laboratory tests may not be performed or the results may be ignored or misplaced. Also, false-positives may occur!

## 11.34  What are the important clinical side-effects that the patient may become aware of with the various disease-modifying drugs?

- *Hydroxychloroquine* can very rarely cause skin rashes and nausea and, exceptionally rarely, retinal damage with visual disturbance.
- *Sulphasalazine* is associated with nausea, skin rashes, abdominal discomfort and occasionally marrow toxicity.
- *Intramuscular gold* can cause skin rashes, mouth ulcers and little else subjectively. For this reason, close attention to the laboratory variables is mandatory.
- *Auranofin*, the oral gold preparation (3 mg daily increasing to 6 mg daily), can cause mild diarrhoea, skin rashes and mouth ulcers and the same laboratory changes as with intramuscular gold but less severely and less frequently.
- *D-penicillamine* may be associated with nausea, skin rashes and a variety of rare entities such as a lupus-like illness, myasthenia gravis, a Goodpasture's-like disease and rare skin disorders. The bone marrow may also be affected.
- *Azathioprine*, too, may cause nausea and general malaise, together with marrow dysfunction.
- *Methotrexate* is associated with alopecia, mouth ulcers, diarrhoea, nausea and the pulmonary toxicity described elsewhere, in addition to rare marrow toxicity.

## 11.35  How best should the GP share care with the rheumatologist?

In general, the GP must get involved and must be primarily in charge of the patient's care. The rheumatologist should be available at the end of the telephone or at the end of a letter, seeing the patient once at the beginning and thereafter perhaps every 6 months or every year, or only if a problem arises. Clearly, it would be impossible for every patient with rheumatoid arthritis to be followed by a rheumatologist. However, it is unnecessary for a rheumatologist to follow such a patient on 3-monthly routine visits but equally inappropriate for a patient to continue from one drug to another in the hands of the GP without ever getting to the rheumatologist. The rheumatologist is in the best position to provide an overall programme of management that will include a multidisciplinary approach to the patient's care.

## PRINCIPLES OF CORTICOSTEROID INJECTION

My advice to GPs is that they should attend an injection clinic (such as the one held at the Royal National Hospital for Rheumatic Diseases in Bath) in order to learn the techniques. A good means of introduction to the subject is to watch the video recently made by the authors — please contact the Royal National Hospital For Rheumatic Diseases (see Appendix 1 for further details).

### 11.36 How often can a joint be injected?

The answer is, as often as necessary, with the proviso that if it needs to be injected more than two or three times per year, another way of managing the problem should be sought. So, in essence, three per year is maximum.

### 11.37 What preparation is used when injecting corticosteroid into a joint, tendosynovial sheath or subperiostally at an insertion of an enthesis?

My approach is to use long-acting corticosteroids, which, in the UK, means triamcinolone hexacetonide or methylprednisolone. Provided that attention is paid to ensuring that there is little or no infiltration of corticosteroid into the subcutaneous tissue, subcutaneous atrophy will not be a problem. For this reason it is always best to infiltrate below the periosteum at, for example, the lateral or medial epicondyle sites.

### 11.38 What local anaesthetic/steroid mixtures are available, and when should they be used?

This is an interesting question given that the package insert on methylprednisolone categorically states that it should not be mixed with lignocaine but most rheumatologists would do so. (Supposedly, the manufacturer is worried about the steroid flocculating in the lignocaine — but this does not seem to occur.) My own approach is always to use the mixture of corticosteroid and lignocaine and there are therefore three possibilities: (1) triamcinolone with added lignocaine; (2) methyl prednisolone/lignocaine mixture, which comes already made up or one can go against the recommendation of the makers; (3) lignocaine added to methylprednisolone.

The advantage of having lignocaine added to the mixture is that there is less discomfort immediately following the procedure on the one hand and an increased volume on the other. For example, when injecting a knee I would use steroid plus 5 ml lignocaine. In those situations where a large volume should be avoided (e.g. injecting the median nerve compartment or the tenosynovial sheath in a patient with a stenosing tenosynovitis or trigger finger) the methylprednisolone/lignocaine mixture is an advantage. The reasons why the pharmaceutical company is anxious for methylprednisolone not to be added to lignocaine is that the former can flocculate and cause technical or aesthetic difficulties. However, many of us are not concerned about the appearance and would go ahead with added lignocaine should we wish a larger volume than that provided with the ready mixed material.

Specifically, methylprednisolone is available at 40 mg in 1 ml alone or 40 mg with lignocaine in 1 ml or 80 mg with lignocaine in 2 ml. However, if I were to inject a knee or a hip, for example, I would want to use 80 mg of methylprednisolone and 5 ml of lignocaine and would therefore add additional material. Alternatively, 40 mg of triamcinolone hexacetonide could be used with 5 ml of lignocaine. Roughly, 20 mg triamcinolone is equivalent to 40 mg methylprednisolone.

## 11.39 When should a local anaesthetic steroid mixture not be used?

I would avoid a large volume of local anaesthetic when injecting in a tenosynovial sheath in a digit or in the carpal tunnel. Personally, I am always happy to use a small amount of anaesthetic but would perhaps use it sparingly in volume with no more than 0.25 ml in certain situations.

## 11.40 When would you use bupivacaine?

Bupivacaine is a long-acting anaesthetic — rarely used in rheumatological practice except, for example, in suprascapular nerve blocks for those with intractable shoulder pain.

## NON-DRUG TREATMENT AND LONG-TERM PATIENT CARE

### 11.41  What should patients be told about the prognosis of chronic rheumatological conditions?

We should always be totally frank with our patients. Often we will not know the prognosis and that must be clearly stated. We can always review the situation a week later or a year later and may then be in a better position to provide them with this important information. Clearly, in some conditions it is very difficult at the outset to know what will happen over the next months and years but even then we should be able to give them an idea about the spectrum, often confidently reassuring them that they are unlikely to be at the bad end. However, for those individuals who clearly are destined to fare badly, it is even more important for us to be absolutely honest lest we lose their confidence — which could result in them ending up in the hands of others less equipped to deal with their problems.

### 11.42  What sort of advice should be given to patients?

Patients want information and advice. In all the social science studies assessing patients' response to their visits to practitioners or rheumatologists, the data show that the chief complaint is lack of information. In addition we know that patients are getting input from their neighbours, family members, other patients, the media, aromatherapists, acupuncturists, osteopaths, chiropractitioners, etc., and not nearly enough from their own physicians. All this has to change. Clearly, in the UK, the great difficulty is that of time, there being only a few minutes per patient in general practice and often little more in rheumatology clinics.

We can somehow alter this by concentrating more on how we conduct our time with our patients and also in providing them with written material. For many specific forms of arthritis there are excellent patient groups such as the National Ankylosing Spondylitis Society or the National Osteoporosis Society (see Appendix 1). These patient-run societies provide excellent information and support for patients. All individuals with a chronic disease and many of those with a self-limiting problem must be given more helpful input from physicians, lest misinformation be soaked up by our patients from all the other sources. The GP and the rheumatologist, together with their teams, must be the patient's advocate and if we fail no one else can take our place.

### 11.43 What can patients with rheumatological disorders do to help themselves?

A great deal. First, it is of paramount importance that they have clear insight into the nature of their disease and the methods of management. Secondly, they should gain most of their information from reliable sources such as the GP or rheumatologist or other members of the health team since much conflicting information will be available to them from neighbours, friends, the media and elsewhere. Confusion is often a major source of anguish for our patients. (See Appendix 1 for useful addresses.)

### 11.44 What allowances are available to these patients?

It is difficult for any practising physician to keep up with the latest legislation regarding allowances for patients. My approach is to identify the patient at need and to involve the Social Services. There is no simple answer given that there is marked geographic variation from city to city and county to county in spite of national legislation.

### 11.45 Where else can the patient turn?

Frequently, the patient can get further advice and help from the Citizens' Advice Bureau, the local church and other local community organization.

### 11.46 Many patients claim that their joints become more painful during damp weather. What is the relationship between climate and symptoms?

This question has vexed clinicians and research workers for decades. Indeed, virtually every patient with an inflammatory disease and many with mechanical joint problems claim that 'bad weather' makes their joints worse and *vice versa*. When this has been studied formally in carefully controlled situations using hermetically sealed cabinets with controlled atmospheric change, no substantiation of the claims could be made. However, many of us feel that the technical conditions were at fault rather than the hypothesis.

Studying the situation worldwide it would appear that it is not 'bad' weather *per se* but rather a falling barometric pressure, which would appear to be related to increasing joint symptoms. This makes sense in terms of what we understand about pressure changes within joints and the inevitable effects on the nerve receptors relating to this change.

It happens that, in the UK, a falling pressure is usually associated with increasing cloud and rain, explaining why patients associate this form of weather with bad joints. Elsewhere in the world a falling barometric pressure can still be associated with clear skies but deteriorating joints.

### 11.47  What should be the aims of shared care?

There is perhaps no other area more suited to shared care than that of managing a patient with chronic rheumatological disease. First, the patient is not living in a vacuum and no one is better equipped to see a patient as a whole person than the GP who will know the family and social situation. However good the rheumatologist, the specialist will only know about the clinical situation second hand, and often information will only be gained from a distance.

In an ideal situation, the family practitioner and rheumatologist will organize a multidisciplinary approach to the management of the patient with chronic disease. Specifically, there should be input from arthritis nurses, physiotherapists, hand therapists and occupational therapists dealing with arthritis care. In addition, patients can get advice from a variety of self-help groups or patient advisory councils (for contact addresses see Appendix 1).

Again, in an ideal situation, the occupational therapist will visit the home with the patient and spouse or partner. By so doing, the needs of the patient can be clearly defined in the specific home setting and advice can then be forthcoming to help with everyday activities of daily living. This may be a simple matter of advice regarding turning on taps, opening jars, getting in and out of a bath etc., or it may require additional appliances to help in dressing and undressing, self-hygiene and activities ranging from cooking to hobbies.

In general, the GP should get involved and must be primarily in charge of the patient's care. The rheumatologist should be available at the end of the telephone or at the end of a letter, seeing the patient once at the beginning and thereafter perhaps every 6 months or every year, or only if a problem arises. Clearly, it would be impossible for every patient with RA to be followed by a rheumatologist. However, it is unnecessary for a rheumatologist to follow up such as patient on 3-monthly routine visits but equally inappropriate for a patient to be changed from one drug to another without ever getting to the rheumatologist. The rheumatologist is in the best position to provide an overall programme of management that will include a multidisciplinary approach to the patient's care.

### 11.48 What modalities are recommended for rehabilitation?

Each patient has to be treated as a unique individual. As intimated above, the therapy may require the entire multidisciplinary team or may be a more structured approach with just physician and a dietician or physician and nurse. Dry land physiotherapy may suffice or hydrotherapy may be indicated. Initially each patient is assessed with these various possibilities in mind and then a programme tailored to the needs of the patient is carried out.

### 11.49 What are the respective roles of the physiotherapist and the occupational therapist?

In general, the physiotherapist looks after the entire body while the occupational therapist focuses on specific functional problems and the ways these can be addressed. For example, a patient with rheumatoid disease may have difficulty with hand function and the occupational therapist will be able to consider the patient in the home or workplace and assess what the patient should be doing for him or herself and what society can do to help the individual. Only by understanding the nature of the clinical problem, the functional status of the patient and the requirements of the patient in terms of managing their household activities or occupational programme can the occupational therapist work out the precise management programme that is needed. Occupational therapists also supply the patient with appropriate splints and other modalities.

The physiotherapist will often be the first person to assess the patient and it may be the physiotherapist who recommends that an occupational therapist should become involved in the patient's care. Usually the home visit would be carried out by the occupational therapist but occasionally the physiotherapist would also be involved.

### 11.50  What practical help is available to patients?

Even more important than specific aids is the general advice about how one can live with the disease: for example, how one should take frequent rests between repetitive jobs, organize one's workday to advantage and use easier work methods with labour-saving appliances, lightweight equipment, long-handled devices to avoid bending and other simple points. Patients are taught about joint protection with simple principles that should be observed:

- Avoid carrying heavy items, where possible, such as shopping bags and trays. A trolley around the house may circumvent some everyday difficulties.
- Use large joints where possible and thus distribute the strain. For example, when carrying a plate use the palm instead of the fingers or use both hands instead of one. Drawers should be shut, for example, with the knee or hip rather than the hand.
- A tight grip should be avoided. The patient should try to avoid using small objects while larger handles can help by simple adaptation.
- Static grip should be avoided. When knitting or holding a book, for example, the book should be rested on a table or book rest and at frequent intervals the fingers should be rested and stretched.
- Finger deviation (ulnar drift) can be avoided to some extent by, for example, using the palm to push oneself up from a chair rather than using the fingers, which will cause further ulnar drift.
- Advice about how to stand, sit, lie when sleeping, lifting, dressing, washing, eating, drinking, shopping and other activities should be given.

There are many simple techniques such as the use of a large-handled peeler for peeling vegetables, a wall-mounted can opener and padding of handles to reduce pressure on the hands. Rather than pouring the contents from a heavy saucepan, a wire chip basket can be placed in the saucepan to cook vegetables and lifted out, draining the fluid, to make the manoeuvre simpler and lighter. Padding the handles of knives and other cooking utensils is also appropriate.

Day splints can be designed as wrist supports and these may increase the functional ability that would otherwise be difficult because of weakness of the wrists. Alternatively, night resting splints may be appropriate to prevent any deformity of the small joints during the night.

## 11.51 Why is complementary medicine so popular with patients?

The choice for the patient is vast. Those who do not like aromatherapy, homeopathy, or herbalists can go to iridopathologists, reflexologists, chiropractitioners or acupuncturists. Then, a third group may wish to follow the naturopath, or a variety of other 'unconventional' remedies.

One criticism levied at practising clinicians is that we fail to make the patient feel comfortable and we fail to talk and listen. There is no doubt that 30 minutes with a herbalist or aromatherapist feels 'better' than a rushed 5-minute interaction with the busy practitioner.

My approach with the patient — particularly those with chronic disease — is to talk about these alternative practitioners. First, I must appear open-minded to the patients and I must gently tell them about the difference between proven and unproved remedies, between those forms of medications that are 'free' under the Health Service and those that are expensive and 'over the counter'. I must also try to listen to patients as well as to talk to them.

I also like to bring in the concept of diet, sooner rather than later. I know that virtually every patient wants to discuss that and they are so anxious lest they forget to raise the point. Indeed, they will often concentrate on nothing that I say until I talk about diet! Again, as tactfully as possible, I point out that some of the worst forms of arthritis that we see are in fish-eating Eskimos or vegetarian groups around the world. Far be it for me to suggest they avoid fish or vegetables but at least the point can be made that there is no such thing as an anti-arthritis diet. Even if there were, one would have to accept that there are some one or two hundred such diets to select from! Clearly, if any really worked we would only need to have *one* anti-arthritis diet!

### 11.52  Do copper bracelets help?

This and other questions relating to alternative therapies are frequently posed by patients. Provided that the modality is neither expensive nor toxic, I am happy to condone such approaches. There is, of course, no scientific evidence to support the use of treatments of this sort.

# 12. The future

Naturally, the rheumatologist's dream is to learn how to prevent disease before it occurs. This requires a major epidemiological exercise with a focus on both the genetic background and the environmental triggers.

The former is a realistic goal. Every practitioner is familiar with the concept of the exploration of the human genome and we are told that by the beginning of the 21st century the entire genetic imprint of the human race will have been defined at a molecular level. At least, in theory, this will allow us to understand more precisely which patient is at risk for which rheumatological disorder. We will then be able to pay attention more precisely to the environmental triggers that are also needed even in the most obviously genetically related disorders. Careful epidemiological study within families, within different ethnic groups, focusing on geographic migration and other epidemiological tools will allow a better understanding of what precipitates disease in those who are most at risk.

In some situations it will become obvious that certain subjects are susceptible to certain infective triggers and the next step would be the development of appropriate vaccinations for such subjects. In addition, other preventive steps are potentially feasible. For example, individuals at risk for 'osteoarthritis' may take a drug prophylactically that would stimulate their cartilage. Indeed, we are beginning to hear of cartilage growth factors that can modulate the effect of the natural downhill process known as 'degenerative joint disease'. It is not unreasonable that within 5–10 years, degenerative arthropathy could be 'modified' or prevented.

For those individuals who still get arthritis, we would hope to be able to recognize earlier in the course of the disease the precise nature of the pathological process. New imaging techniques are arriving on a monthly basis. Sixth- or seventh-generation MRI scanners and isotope scanning with isotopes that recognize and target special tissues are becoming available and many other innovative processes will allow early localization and recognition of pathological sites.

Our treatment modalities will become tailor-made both to the individual and to the specific pathological process. It is not unreasonable to assume that, as we understand more about the genetic profile of the patient, safer agents will be available on a custom-made basis, thus preventing some of the more toxic reactions when one drug is given to many different people of different genetic backgrounds. As the agent can become targeted not only for the individual but also for the relevant tissue, there should be fewer systemic side-effects and greater efficacy. For example, newer NSAIDs, which are type 2 cyclo-oxygenase-specific may have less impact on the gastro-protective cyclo-oxygenases than the older, non-specific type 1 cyclo-oxygenase inhibitors.

There will be developments in both the non-steroidals and disease-modifying agents. Tenidap is a new and interesting drug that is due to come onto the market in 1996. It has both NSAID and disease-modifying characteristics. In theory, patients with rheumatoid arthritis should require only tenidap rather than an NSAID plus a second-line agent.

Although it would be naive to think that all 220 forms of rheumatological disease will disappear in the next century, it is at least reasonable to anticipate that there should be much less suffering in the relatively near future.

Finally, it is worth looking back at the last 100 years. There is no doubt that some of the major destructive arthropathies are now historical remnants. For example, some of the great infective arthropathies have largely melted away in the Western world. As the specific virus (retrovirus?) becomes defined in, for example, the aetiology of rheumatoid disease, we will anticipate antiviral agents that will be capable of curing rheumatoid arthritis in the same way that penicillin can 'cure' rheumatic fever. The goal must be that the major chronic rheumatic diseases of the end of the 20th century will become short-lived, self-limiting, annoying problems as the 21st century begins.

# Appendix 1: Useful addresses

National Osteoporosis Society
PO Box 10
Radstock
Bath BA3 3YB
Tel: 01761-432472

Arthritis Care
18 Stephenson Way
London NW1 2HD
Tel: 0171-916-1500

The Arthritis & Rheumatism Council
Copeman House
St Mary's Court
St Mary's Gate
Chesterfield
Derbyshire S41 7TD
Tel: 01246-558033

National Ankylosing Spondylitis
Society
5 Grosvenor Crescent
London SW1X 7ER
Tel: 0171-630-6384

Lupus UK
Queens Court
9-17 Eastern Road
Romford
Essex RM1 3NG
Tel: 01708-731251

Royal National Hospital for
Rheumatic Diseases
Upper Borough Walls
Bath BA1 1 RL
Tel: 01225-465941
Fax: 01225-421202

(Regarding injection clinics, rheumatological teaching clinics, injection
videos etc.)

Primary Care Rheumatology Society
55 South Parade
North Allerton
North Yorkshire DL7 8SL
Tel: 01609-774794

# Appendix 2: Guidelines for the monitoring of disease-modifying anti-rheumatic drugs

| Drug | Baseline and monitoring tests | Frequency of tests | Values requiring action | Action |
|---|---|---|---|---|
| Sulphasalazine (up to 3g/day) | Full blood count | Monthly for 3 months, then 3-monthly | Platelets ↓ WBC ↓ | Stop, recheck restart possibly at lower dose |
| Gold injections (up to 50 mg weekly) | Full blood count | Monthly, then 2–3-monthly | As for sulphasalazine | As for sulphasalazine |
| | Urinalysis | With each injection | Proteinuria 2+ | Check MSU, 24-hour protein, *renal function, check FBC |
| Oral gold (up to 9 mg daily) | Full blood count | Monthly, then 2–3-monthly after 2 g | As for sulphasalazine | As for sulphasalazine |
| | Urinalysis | Monthly | | |
| D-penicillamine (125–750 mg daily) | Full blood count Urinalysis *Renal function } | Monthly | As for sulphasalazine | As for sulphasalazine |
| Methotrexate (up to 20 mg weekly) | Full blood count | After 2 weeks initially, monthly for 3/12, then 6–8 weeks | As for sulphasalazine | As for sulphasalazine |
| | Liver function | 4–12 weekly | ALT 3× normal | Stop, recheck, restart at lower dose |
| Azathioprine (up to 2.5 mg/kg daily) | Full blood count | Monthly | As for sulphasalazine | As for sulphasalazine. Stop, recheck, urinalysis. MSU |
| Hydroxy-chloroquine (up to 400 mg daily for 3 months then 200 mg daily) | No ophthalmic, haematological, biochemical or urinary monitoring required, assess eye status only | | | |

*Renal function indicated by urea, creatinine and creatinine clearance.

# Index